# THE HOT MOMMY'S SECRET

## FITNESS, FOOD & ATTITUDE

By Holly Chisholm Hargrave

## DISCLAIMER

This book is not intended to treat, diagnose or prescribe. The information contained herin is in no way to be considered as a substitute for a consultation with a duly licensed health care professional.

Cover photo: Maggie Marguerite Studios
Cover design: Sally Rinehart
Design & Page Layout: Janzel Martínez

First Edition, 2015
Printed in the United States of America

ISBN-13: 978-0615716206
ISBN-10: 0615716202

Published by:
AthleticGenius LLC
695 Bloomfield Avenue, Montclair, NJ 07042
website: athleticgenius.com email: info@athleticgenius.com

# DEDICATION

*Dedicated, with love, to my children—Holden, Ava, and Hudson—who inspire me every day to demonstrate health, gratitude, and well-being.*

# CONTENTS

# PREFACE

People who meet me often assume I've been athletic my entire life. In fact, they assume that I have always been the picture of health. But the fact is before I became a fitness professional, I was not fit at all. I only became athletic in my late twenties and a dedicated athlete in my mid-thirties.

When I was two years old, I was in a terrifying accident. My brother was cutting our lawn on a riding mower. I wanted a ride on the mower, so I ran to catch up with my brother. At that very moment, he put the tractor into reverse, not realizing I was right behind him. Before he realized what was happening, the tractor had run over my left leg up to my waist!

Not wanting to waste a moment waiting for an ambulance, my parents opted to drive me to the local emergency room themselves. We lived in the suburbs outside Boston, so a surgeon was rushed from the city to my local hospital. The lawn tractor blades amputated my left big toe. My left leg was broken in three places, including the femur, and I had multiple gaping wounds and severed muscles. The doctors weren't confident I would keep my leg due to the contaminants from the lawn tractor. My parents were told I would never walk properly due to the loss of the toe and severity of the bone and muscle damage.

I did not lose my leg, but I had trouble walking as a child and could not participate in normal childhood sports. Dragging a full-leg cast around, I was adamant about keeping up to play with other kids. This tenacity was my saving grace. The overall effects of the accident were the loss of my big toe, a one-eighth-inch difference in leg length, and permanently severed leg muscles. Even today, the loss of a big toe alone will disqualify a person from enlisting in the military. The big toe takes 40 percent of the body's gait weight load. Not surprisingly, the loss of my big toe has been the most challenging to overcome. The big toe affects everything right up the body chain from the foot to the ankle, calf, hips, lower back, and directly to the shoulder. Its loss impedes the ability to run long distances and lessens the ability to run fast.

Even today, digit and limb amputation is common in our society where obesity is an epidemic. Obesity-induced diabetes mellitus, or type 2 diabetes, can cause circulation problems in 10.4 percent of the U.S. population.[1] Nerve disease and decreased circulation can cause cell death and the need for a toe amputation. That unfortunate procedure can lead to the imbalances I suffered. Physical therapy becomes necessary to rebuild strength, balance, and coordination.

Not surprisingly, dysfunctional anatomical patterns came from the loss of my big toe. I took action to help my body healthily compensate to correct my balance. In order to make up for my anatomical compensation, as an adult, I strengthened gluteal, knee, and leg muscles.

My muscle weakness and awkward gait made it painful to participate in most sports due to inflammation. Unable to participate in school sports due to pain and weakness, I was the kid in gym class by the bleachers doing physical therapy. Physical therapy at that time (and still today), couldn't totally cure a nine-toed gait. However, it has advanced incredibly over the last forty-plus years.

[1] http://www.cdc.gov/diabetes/pubs/statsreport14/national-diabetes-report-web.pdf

Back then, my therapy was limited to using a resistance band to perform leg extension exercises.

Fast-forward to my early career in the pharmaceutical industry. My first job was an area anesthesia specialist in sales management. In this role, I taught anesthesiologists how to utilize various drugs and equipment in the operating room to manage patients having surgery under either local or general anesthesia. Being there allowed me to see every muscle and organ in the human body.

The connection of all the joints and muscles of the body began to make sense for me. It became apparent that my missing toe caused a chain reaction throughout my body, and I needed to focus on many muscles to correct the loss. I embarked on an exercise program to strengthen my leg, gluteus, back, and shoulder muscles.

Gradually, I got stronger and was able to exercise more than I ever had in my life. Working out significantly reduced my pain from inflammation caused by my off-balanced gait and weak muscles. It also improved my balance. My injuries still affect me today. They make it more challenging to perform my jobs as a fitness instructor and a mom. I use a lot of ice; however, I am convinced that if I did not choose to stay strong, the pain of being sedentary would be far worse and would prevent me from playing sports with my children.

The fact is that muscles are more critical to our ability to function than most of us imagine. We think of muscles as tools for strength only. But the 650 muscles of the body are involved in all of our daily functions: walking, talking, sitting, standing, eating, and even breathing. Muscles also help to maintain posture, circulate blood, and protect the organs.

In life's journey, little did I know how important becoming fit would be for my family. One day, I was pushing my youngest child, Hudson, in a stroller. At a street crossing, we stopped and waited for the traffic to clear. The traffic stopped and a kind gentleman in the first car waiting patiently at the crosswalk waved at us to go ahead and cross the street. I checked in all directions and walked forward. When we were in the middle of the street, a driver turned through a blinking red light and hit us head-on. Hudson's stroller went flying, and I ended up on the windshield of the car. The driver stopped, and I fell off the car, landing in the middle of the street. I reacted as any mother would and got up and ran to find my baby. I was terrified to think he was lying in the middle of the street in imminent danger.

Thankfully, an off-duty officer was behind the car that struck us. He reacted by quickly picking up my son and carrying him out of the street. I yelled at him to give me my baby. He showed me his badge and said, "You'd better sit down."

It was only then that I realized what a shaking mess I was, with cuts and abrasions all over. Hudson and I spent seven hours in the emergency room that afternoon and into the evening. The doctors and nurses who treated me said that if I had not been so fit, my bones likely would have broken. They also told me that being physically active had given me the reaction time and balance to manage the impact of the car.

My recovery began with walking, then walk/jogging, and finally jogging. Four years later, as of this writing, I am back to a seven-minute mile for the duration of a thirteen-mile run. I share this story so you understand that it is important to know that as we age, balance becomes more and more critical, and keeping fit should include honing balance. If I was able to recover from such an injury, so can you achieve your goals.

Do you have to run a seven-minute mile? Hell no! Set a personal standard that makes you happy and represents balance in your life. Pursue that standard with pride and passion.

As for my diet: did I grow up eating healthy? No way! I grew up on Tab brand diet soda and frozen dinners. My mother was not a cook. As a treat, she would make us white bread slathered with Crisco and sprinkled with refined sugar. Over the years, I have educated myself about proper nutrition and have changed my way of eating. I revel in the energetic feeling I can achieve through eating smart. I wish I could give you the gift of experiencing just how amazing it feels, physically and mentally, to exercise and eat right.

We live busy lives, and as a result, often adjust to living in a state of health mediocrity. Mediocrity becomes our norm. I wrote this book to enable you to change your personal standard. Fitness is a journey, not a destination. You don't arrive there and stop. I work every day to model fitness and health to my clients, children, and those who surround me. My secret is vigilance and self-awareness. My hope is that my strategies will help you attain your goals in a way that is sustainable in your lifestyle so that you will feel empowered by energy and self-confidence.

I wrote The Hot Mommy's Secret to help you reach your health and fitness goals. I've done the hard work in my own life to achieve a healthy lifestyle, and I'd like to share my secrets with you so that you can be your personal best. Exercising and eating healthy can be difficult, especially getting started or restarted after having children. Your kids may even encourage the battle against eating healthy by protesting vegetables, fruits, and healthy foods. Everyone has to start somewhere. That mom you see with the great body had to change her eating habits and do her first sit-up.

The secret is simple: focus on your wellness by using the tools I will share in this book to be the best you that you can be!

Let's get moving!

# INTRODUCTION

Moms are typically the central coordinators of any family. Nimble and expert at multitasking, we tend to be the ones creating order out of chaos. We somehow manage to clean up the breakfast mess, call our moms, change the kitty litter, and pack three lunches, all just before darting off to a business meeting or whatever our next obligation might be. According to a recent study, two-thirds of mothers say they are multitasking nearly every waking minute. Many admitted to cleaning the shower while bathing in it, and cooking dinner while coloring their hair.[2] Personally, I admit to eating my chicken wrap by taking a big bite and scarfing it down while in the shower! We mothers certainly get things done, but often at the cost of caring for ourselves. My mission is to urge you to prioritize your own health and fitness and guide you in how to do it. Everything else—inner peace and family cohesion, most importantly—depends on your physical and mental well-being. Lots of books discuss how to "self-love." I hope you will find this book different because I intend to make the concept your "reality."

The challenges of motherhood begin immediately when you become pregnant. Morning sickness and exhaustion at the end of the day will likely affect both your diet and

---

[2] Deni Kirkova, "Rise of the Superhuman Mums," *Daily Mail*, March 25, 2013, http://www.dailymail.co.uk/femail/article-2298347/Supermums-Two-thirds-mothers-admit-multi-tasking-EVERY-waking-hour-new-survey-reveals.html

exercise routine. Whether you had an established exercise program prior to pregnancy or would like to establish a new one, consult your physician to obtain exercise approval and guidance. Being pregnant can be a great time to get your body moving, even if you have not exercised in recent memory. Some of the many benefits of exercise during pregnancy include:

- Good mood as a result of "feel-good" brain endorphins
- Increased energy
- Prevention of unnecessary weight gain
- Better sleep patterns

Be careful! Water retention and loosening of joints during pregnancy can make your grip less firm and cause a shift in your center of gravity. Lack of dexterity and clumsiness is common during pregnancy. Exercise with caution and save those agility sports for post-pregnancy. Remember, pregnancy only lasts for nine months. During those months, proceed with caution for you and your baby. Be sure to monitor your exertion level by listening to your body. If you feel fatigued, rest.

If you belong to a gym or regularly attend a fitness class, advise your instructors immediately of your pregnancy. Your physician will provide you with exercise guidelines to follow during your pregnancy. Your fitness instructor can help you to monitor your exercise to ensure that you remain within those safety guidelines. As accredited and certified instructors, it is their job to be responsible for you. A fitness instructor is required to carry proper certifications and insurance in order to be qualified to teach. Don't be afraid to ask your instructor if he or she has relevant certifications to instruct you during pregnancy. Instructor certifications require continuing education credits (CECs) to be maintained via approved industry testing. Be sure that your instructor has maintained their current accreditations.

# 1

# Where Are My Jeans?

*Hollyism: "There is no shame in being in the process of getting where you want to be, and a lot of glory in having the courage to try."*

This book is for moms with kids of all ages, but let's visit where it all began. Hooray, I...uh, WE...are pregnant! Where is the "we" in that statement? It is *your* body, not your partner's! Joking aside, I was in my mid-thirties when I had my first child, Holden. After months of peeing on ovulation sticks and propping my ass up on pillows post-sex to give the sperm a downhill swim, pregnancy was more like, "Finally!"

I went from thinking, "Now I can't have a glass of wine with dinner," quickly to, "Damn, I am suffering from morning sickness so badly I don't even want to look at a glass of wine." Walking by the seafood department at the grocery store made me gag. I stealthily ducked into the side aisle more than once to vomit into my handbag. I thought to myself, "Wasn't I supposed to be *glowing*, not *growing*, so quickly?" I was sick as a dog and could only keep down crackers. Ah yes, the carbohydrate challenge immediately entered during the first trimester of pregnancy. The carbs I had so carefully avoided became a staple. The entire box of crackers became my new best friend on the side table by my bed at night. Eating crackers while lying in bed would have normally been highly prohibited. I am here to tell you that crackers and ginger ale at bedside are acceptable in nausea crises—and I label massive vomiting as a crisis.

At the end of my pregnancy, I became so uncomfortable that I couldn't wait to get that baby out of my belly! I clearly remember the last days of pregnancy and my inability to see my own feet. I lay in bed in the morning having to pee so badly I pondered the concept of getting out of bed. Perhaps I could tie a rope to the end of my bed to hoist myself up to the toilet without peeing my pants.

Showering and shaving my legs was a feat in itself as I attempted to reach over my huge tummy and catch a glimpse of my unreachable shins and thighs. Months after childbirth, I found unshaven areas I could have woven into proper dreadlocks!

The glorious day that I was to give birth to my bundle of joy finally arrived. I went to the hospital dressed in maternity clothes with my favorite jeans optimistically packed in my suitcase. I was expecting to slip my jeans on for the ride home. Kudos to those who were able to zip their jeans up after giving birth. Clearly, in my case, there was a mix-up; these were someone else's jeans, because I was nowhere close to fitting into this unforgiving pair. Jeans at knee-height, I glanced at the dirty maternity clothes I wore into the hospital still lying on the chair in my room. Feeling a pang of disappointment, I picked them up and slowly slipped them on for the drive home.

This is common and real for most moms, so please do not feel at all disappointed in what you wear home from delivering your bundle of joy. Focus on the magic of the beautiful baby in your arms and be content.

# 2

# Hot Mommy Is Home

*Hollyism: "Everyone's life is unique."*

Once you have your baby, you begin adjusting to motherhood. You may notice that despite no longer carrying a baby around inside you, you still weigh twenty pounds more than you've ever weighed in your life. Those pre-mommy jeans, now buried deep in the bottom dresser drawer, are calling out to you. You wonder if you'll ever be able to get them on and actually zip them up again.

Meanwhile, television shows and magazines feature celebrity mommies who still look slim and fit even while pregnant. These same celebrity moms also lose baby weight in record time and are dubbed "mom-shells." (Get it? Rhymes with bombshells.) As celebrities, it is their job to look fit and fabulous. The pressure on celebrities to appear on the red carpet and before the paparazzi looking fit is unspeakable. But guess what? The National Institute for Health and Clinical Excellence warns that "celebrity claims of unrealistic rapid weight loss" put women under additional pressure at an already stressful time.

In my clients, I commonly see that there is heightened pressure for women to "bounce back" from pregnancy body form. But before I elaborate, let's define the "celebrity mom." These are women who have people who cook their meals, do their laundry and dishes, and clean their houses. They have the time to exercise four hours a day with top-notch personal trainers. In other words, they have the time and budget required to achieve rapid weight loss. While it's nearly impossible to get the same rapid results without personal chefs, trainers, and stylists, it hasn't stopped many regular moms from trying. It's part of a recent trend to lose pregnancy weight faster than ever. Comparing a normal post-pregnancy body to a celeb's is like expecting to be live photo-shopped. Remember, magazine photos are often airbrushed and photoshopped to reflect beyond realistic expectations.[3]

Yet, the pressure trickles down via media images to us regular people and often causes us to judge ourselves harshly. And we, in turn, sometimes allow our insecurities to affect our attitudes toward one another. The result is a bit of a competition to see who can get fit the fastest. Suddenly, we are now comparing ourselves not only to celebrity moms, but also to one another. Which mom is still chubby and who is physically perfect fastest is typically a major topic of conversation. It's good to be aware of this so that you can stop yourself from engaging in comparisons.

Be assured that losing the extra pounds you gained during pregnancy will take time. Don't compare yourself to others, crash diet, and certainly do not engage in "negative self-talk." Be as patient with yourself as you are with your newborn. Right about now, you may be asking, "Who is Holly

[3] http://www.telegraph.co.uk/health/healthnews/7263701/Celebrity-mothers-put-women-under-pressure-to-lose-babyweight-too-fast-Nice.html

to be telling me this?" Holly is a fitness expert, which has provided her with an unfair advantage of being fit for a living. "How could she possibly relate to what every mom goes through, given her career?" Meet Holly; through three pregnancies, I lost and gained a grand total of 150 pounds. I was far from what the media would deem a "mom-shell." I remember, prior to ever being pregnant, looking at expecting women who were in amazing shape in the gym and thinking, "Damn, I hope I look like that when I am pregnant," and realizing, "Damn, I don't look like that now *not* pregnant. How will I possibly look that way pregnant?" Moms are all wired to want the best for our families, and we translate that to our personal best self, physically and mentally. The degrees to which we are self-critical, however, vary. We all share a tendency to be more critical of ourselves than we are of anyone else in our world. Except, of course, should you have a mother-in-law.

An experience I would like to share with you that prompted this book is my feeling of always being in a scramble—disheveled and exhausted. This was the feeling of a mommy life, and in my mind I was mediocre. Motherhood appeared effortless for other women. Clearly, there was something wrong with me.

One day, I arrived to pick up my kids from school in sweaty gym clothes and sneakers. I was late today, yet again, and of course, in a torrential downpour. Out my car window, I saw the most amazing and intimidating sight: a perfectly-dressed, hair done, make-up flawless (strike one) mom who is on time, sporting the perfect umbrella (strike two, ouch) and perfectly-worn blue jeans that look fabulous on her cute behind (strike three—I am so OUT).

Time shifted into slow motion in my mind, and I visualized the school sidewalk becoming her personal fashion show runway. The music began as she gingerly tucked her child under her arm and strolled to her car without a hair out of place. Meanwhile, I got soaked in the downpour, running like a mother duck to gather my three ducklings. I felt so frustrated that I wanted to jam that perfect umbrella up her adorable a**... You get the picture. Sitting drenched in my car with the furious wiper blades swiping back and forth, I gripped my steering wheel in utter frustration.

I had succumbed to this ridiculous mommy competition, and in doing so, served only to make myself feel utterly inadequate. I took a deep breath and silently asked myself, "Why can't I be the perfect hot mom like her? What the hell is she doing that I am not?" Then I realized, it is not about others, it is about me—about my perception of myself.

Be aware that as a mom your perception of yourself is modeled by your children; don't negative self-talk in front of them. Embrace your magnificence. Radiate your self-confidence. When I compliment most moms, they defer the compliment by replying, "I need to lose ten pounds," or, "My thighs are big and my stomach never looked like this." I hope that by the end of reading this book, you will smile at a compliment and simply say, "Thank you." That has been an extremely hard lesson for me to learn in my own life, and I want to impart the ability to recognize your accomplishments rather than focus on your perceived shortcomings. Your children will model your behavior. What do you wish to teach them?

Time to talk the true secrets to being a fit and healthy Hot Mommy. I am going to share the Hot Mommy's Secret with you in this book and hold nothing back. Forget your

15-Minute Abs. Get past your belly-slimming electro belts. Forget sprinkling fairy dust on your food so it magically won't stick to your insides, but instead pass right through, as some miracle products claim. Losing baby weight and staying fit with the demands of motherhood is hard work, but you're more than capable. Exhaustion brought on by the demands of motherhood creates poor eating habits. The schedule of being a mom limits the time we have to prioritize exercise. It may sound cliché, but it's the truth: moms are at the center of every family. We are cornerstones of our home, and we manage to keep it in mechanical—and on some days, mania-cal—order. We manage to clean up after a torrential breakfast of leftovers before we dart off to our next obligation. Women constantly execute from multiple angles. We are masters at adapting to accommodate the demands of motherhood.

# 3

# Post-Baby Booty

*Hollyism: "Embrace change."*

When adjusting to motherhood, you will experience a realm of physical and emotional changes. Welcome to crying at greeting cards, heart-wrenching social media posts, and living in pajamas. Hopefully you will not experience postpartum depression. (If you do, you need a different book and to consult your physician immediately.) You may notice that despite no longer carrying a baby around inside you, you still weigh twenty pounds more than your pre-pregnancy weight. Meanwhile, those pre-mommy jeans buried deep in the bottom dresser drawer are calling you. How do you move yourself toward zipping them up again? Let me get you started with some healthy advice regarding what you can expect from your body post pregnancy.

Body changes after childbirth can include:
- Your body composition can shift
- The way fat is redistributed in your body can change
- Your shoe size can change
- Your breast size can change

- Your hair may become straight or curly or change texture.[4]

During pregnancy, your body composition can shift. It is realistic that you won't return back to the exact pre-pregnancy weight and shape. Initially your body weight being beyond your baby's actual birth weight is perfectly normal. Frankly, things—like your internal organs—get temporarily relocated. Relocation takes time for adjustment, be it physical or geographical.

Every woman will react differently to the effects of pregnancy and childbirth. Much depends upon fatigue, nutrition, and method of childbirth—C-section, episiotomy or tear, long labor, etc. Pregnancy and childbirth have a tendency to cause a number of minor health problems including but not limited to:

- Back pain
- Hemorrhoids
- Constipation
- Varicose veins

The most important thing to remember is that the postpartum period is a time of transition during which we must take care of ourselves. The first six weeks are a time of healing and recovery. It takes the genital organs six to eight weeks to return to their original size and function. The pregnancy hormone relaxin, which increases the size and elasticity of connective tissues (ligaments and muscles), will remain in a new mother's body for up to five months. This is why a new mother's joints are so fragile (50 percent of them

---

[4] Tracee Cornforth, "What Women Need to Know About Post Pregnancy: How to Have an Easy Post-Pregnancy Period," *About Health*, January 29, 2008, http://womenshealth.about.com/cs/pregnancy/a/postpregbook.htm

experience back pain) and why any high-impact activity puts tremendous stress on the pelvic floor and the abdominal organs. Frankly, this is why you pee during jumping jacks!

Pregnancy changes a woman's body—sometimes forever. Some of the resulting shifts are less welcome than others, but consider them phenomenal. You have just created a baby—a life that will last for many years of joy. Below, I will review a few changes that can last at least six months but could become permanent.

**Hair loss and/or change in texture.** Many moms may lose their hair. You will find piles of it in the shower drain. Some do get their thickness back, but others will end up with thinner hair. My last baby, Hudson, literally curled my hair. I went from jet straight hair to curly hair. Too bad it's not still the eighties; he would have saved me money on perms!

**Boobs.** You may easily lose up to a cup size in your breasts. This has to do with both pregnancy and breastfeeding. You may find they get a little saggy or a tad bit smaller. I went from a 36D to a 34A.

**Feet.** Your feet will get bigger. I have gone from a size seven and a half to a size nine. This has to do with fluid retention during pregnancy, but can result in a permanent increase in shoe size.

**Body Composition.** Your overall shape may change. You might find that you never had hips, and now you do. Perhaps your tummy was always flat, and now you gather weight there. Consider these body shifts voluptuous and understand that with exercise and proper nutrition, you will love your post-baby body.

Finding the time to fit in important exercise and proper nutrition will be a challenge. Children, especially babies, are adorable in the most life-altering way, however extremely demanding of our time. Faced with the limitation of only twenty-four hours in a day, you may be tempted to try to find shortcuts to getting fit.

Don't fall for ads from hucksters who want to take advantage of the combination of our vanity and lack of time. Losing baby weight and staying fit with the demands of motherhood is hard work. But you're more than capable.

You may initially find losing weight a challenge. For one thing, you'll likely be sleep-deprived caring for the baby. Sleep deprivation can result in eating poorly just to stay awake. When we are overtired, we tend to make poor food choices. This is because we seek rapid sugar energy via simple carbs and sweets. And, of course, the schedule of caring for a baby limits the amount of time we have to exercise. Here are four important tips for staying reasonably fit and healthy while caring for a baby:

**Tip 1:** Be sure to eat breakfast. Breakfast should contain a combination of protein and complex carbohydrates.

**Tip 2:** Eat small, high-protein, low-sugar, low-fat, low-sodium meals about every three hours to maintain consistent blood sugar levels. This will help you maintain consistent energy levels.

**Tip 3:** Learn to nap when the baby naps. Sleep deprivation causes you to reach for a quick source of energy—foods containing simple sugars. These contain high sugar and simple carbohydrate content.

**Tip 4:** Don't be shy about asking for help. Ask your spouse to feed the baby once per night so you can get a full six hours of sleep. Then get up early and exercise while the baby and your spouse are sleeping. Also, exercise when your spouse is available to watch the baby, and plan your rest and eating accordingly so that you are best prepared to utilize your time efficiently rested and fueled.

When your spouse isn't available, find a friend or family member who can offer you an hour of babysitting a day so that you can exercise. Do not be hesitant. Most people understand how exhausting it is to be a new mom. People will want to help and will feel honored that you would entrust them with your beautiful child. It is important to not give in to the temptation to use your free time to tidy up or run errands. Your physical and mental well-being is more important.

# 4

# Nothing to Lose, Everything to Gain

*Hollyism: "You have more freedom than you're using. Don't constrain your health and wellness by using errands or other obligations as excuses. Prioritize fitness."*

Getting motivated is the first step toward fitness. You are able, but you must be willing. You have the strength, passion, and ability to achieve your goals. Decide you're no longer willing to stay where you are and engage your amazing ability to move forward. Motivation and organization are the first steps toward getting fit. I happen to have a few tricks to guide you to success.

In order to get motivated, create a vision board. Purchase a poster board and glue onto it photos and quotations that inspire you to get moving and eating right. Choose photos from your past—a time when you looked the way you want to look again—as well as your aspired future. Visualization is powerful, and the images should reflect your ideal of happiness. Search books, magazines, and the Internet. Seek images not of mom-shells, but of those with an emotional impact such as beach, sunset, mountains, healthy foods, or fitness photos. Any image that makes you feel inspired will work. Next, choose sayings that inspire you and add them to your image board.

Alternatively, you could use a mental image to hold in awareness as you exercise. Losing the fifty pounds of weight I put on with my last child, Hudson, was beyond difficult for me. As I was caring for my two toddlers as well as my newborn, exhaustion had me incoherent. I needed a mental image to inspire me. What worked for me was imagining myself wearing a backpack filled with forty-five pounds worth of my children's favorite books, equal to forty-five pounds in body weight. I promised myself I would eat right and exercise enough to remove one book from the backpack each week until I finally made it to my original weight. It was painful and took almost a year, but it worked! Find your motivation, be it visual, mental, or a combination of the two. Every journey is unique because you are amazingly unique.

Get organized. Begin each day with a list of priorities, and ask yourself, "If 'x' doesn't get done, what will happen? Will the world end?" Divide your day into two categories: "Must To-Do" and "Optional To-Do." At first, write comprehensive decision-making lists. After a short time, these lists will become part of your cerebral process and will no longer need to be written in detail.

The Optional To-Do list represents your barriers to motivation. They distract you and steal your energy, preventing you from obtaining your healthy lifestyle by eating smart, exercising, and getting proper rest. We all fall victim to that one toy left on the floor, dirty sock that fell out of the hamper, or dirty dish in the sink. Teach yourself to only see the Must

To-Do things in order to keep yourself focused, organized, and on track to success.

This is not easy when you have lived in a pre-baby, organized environment. Tripping over shoes makes your blood pressure spike, and stepping on a pile of goo on the floor is no fun. Let me provide you some Hot Mommy's Little Secrets to prioritize your daily organization.

### Must To-Do: What needs to get done?

- Basic groceries (not for a snowstorm or hurricane)
- Diapers must be changed
- Feed the family
- Necessary laundry
- Exercise
- Household bills

### Optional To-Do: What won't cause the world to end?

- Prepare gourmet meals
- Last load of laundry must be washed
- Closet organization
- Laundry folded
- Match socks from laundry (tormenting)
- Keep the family car pristine (it will get messy)

Tackle the daily challenges with organization. Losing keys? Always keep them in the same place, like by the phone. Constantly tripping over shoes? Get an inexpensive crate to throw them in for short term. Baskets and inexpensive storage bins can also help you organize the most troublesome items in your life. As for tasks, having a rough idea of when you'll tackle them can give you a sense of calm throughout the week. For example, do laundry on Sunday mornings, pay bills on Wednesdays, and so on. Have a schedule so you won't feel your blood pressure rise trying to cram a million tasks into already jam-packed days.

Smooth out the bumps in your mommy mornings. Mornings are exceptionally rough for moms. Sleep deprivation makes the entire process become exponentially harder when you have to wake, feed, dress, and potentially pack for and transport a small child in addition to yourself for a workout at your gym. Here are some ideas for helping you take control of your mornings despite all the challenges involved.

Do as much as you possibly can the night before. Set out clothes for the next day, both for yourself and for your child. Make sure diaper bags are ready to go. Wake up before your child does to have a cup of coffee, get dressed, and take care of your own breakfast before baby gets moving. Once baby wakes, you'll feel less crazed and more able to focus your attention, which equals organization and motivation. Ideally, choose an exercise or fitness activity that is close to home. Finally, make friends with other parents who may be able to give your kids rides to activities when you can't. Be sure to return the favor in ways that fit into your schedule.

# 5
# G.P.S.—Goals, Performance, Success

*Hollyism: "Define your destination."*

If you don't know where you are going, even that darling Siri can't help you arrive at your destination. You must determine your personal goals. Setting goals is critical in your journey toward a lifetime of fitness. The first step is to define your personal goals by making a list that is realistic, achievable, and sustainable. Remember, in setting your goals, do not set unrealistic goals; this will only result in disappointment. A secret to accomplishing your goals is committing to them by writing them down on paper or saving them on your computer, as long as the tool allows you to document progress toward your goals in a reviewable format.

Written and visual goals are powerful because writing down your goals forces you to select something specific and define clearly what you want to achieve. Goals that are not measurable cannot translate into results.

Written goals also aid in prioritization of goals via requiring articulation and intention to achieve your goals. By writing down your goals, you are creating a "contract" with yourself to take action toward achievement. In the daily deluge of motherhood responsibilities, written goals will remind you to prioritize yourself. Consider it a contract with yourself.

Written goals support your motivation to overcome obstacles. Effort for change will create resistance. Good change or bad change is change. Change is difficult. From the moment you set a goal, you will begin to feel the obstacles. Do not focus on the dynamics of the obstacles; doing this will only give them power to prevent your success. Take your power back by reviewing your written goals. Only when you see your obstacles can you create a strategy to overcome them.

Documented goals help celebrate progress. Motherhood is challenging. Some days, you may feel like you are just not making any progress. Some days, you actually may not be, but that is okay too. Revisiting your written goals may surprise you by what you have achieved. We can get so focused on where we are going that we forget how far we have already come.

**Key example goals:**
- Goal 1: Lose the baby weight.
- Goal 2: Resume an exercise program or start one for the first time.
- Goal 3: Increase energy level.
- Goal 4: Feel emotionally and physically healthier.

To get organized and make progress toward your goals, my secret weapon is my daily journal. To write on its pages makes me feel accountable. I like a nice journal sitting on my desk, counter, or dresser. I prefer paper instead of electronic, but one size doesn't fit all when it comes to technology. You might prefer to use your computer, smartphone, or other device. Just make sure that whatever it is looks at you with puppy eyes during your day and can't be ignored.

In your Hot Mommy Journal, you will keep track of:

- What you eat
- Why you eat (hunger, fatigue, stress, etc.)
- Weight and/or body measurements
- Exercise routine
- Sleep patterns

What you eat includes tracking your eating patterns by documenting what time you ate and what you ate throughout the day, including portion sizes, to the best of your memory. Review this data to note good food choices, bad food choices, any times that you did not eat breakfast, or any time you fasted longer than three hours during the day. Remember to note water intake; target eight, eight-ounce glasses per day.

Why you eat includes your emotional feelings toward food. Note if you overate and why. It is important that when writing in your journal to note things such as your mood. For example:

- "I was feeling raging hormones and major anxiety."
- "I was stressed at work or home, and overtired."
- "As a result of stress, I ate an entire bag of chips and an ice cream sandwich, and washed it all down with a bottle of Chardonnay."

Emotional eating is very common. Feeling stressed and eating food for comfort to assist you in calming down is a quick fix many of us utilize. Also note the time you eat, which will show you the length of time you sometimes go without eating properly. This will reveal if perhaps you are skipping meals, and as a result of under-eating during the day are over-snacking at night.

Understanding your eating patterns will enable you to make better decisions for yourself as you move forward.

Weight and/or body measurements include a record of your baseline information related to your size, body composition, and body weight. This baseline will be needed in order to measure results. Baseline means current measurements. Record your baseline weight, and weigh yourself on a consistent schedule at the same time each day or week. What interval is best to weigh yourself, daily, weekly, or monthly? The simple answer is whatever works best for you, but never, ever more than once per day. Be aware that there are ups and downs from day to day due to water weight and many other things. If you find the scale becoming discouraging, cut down on the frequency of weighing in; negative feedback is not what you are seeking. Unless you have a very advanced scale that offers data including age, body mass index, water weight, and muscle mass, it is a variable measurement. Most scales are in bathrooms and most bathrooms have windows. In case of emergency, look out below—falling scale! If the number on the scale causes you stress, don't use it. Instead, use either your measurements or a "test outfit."

To take your measurements, use a soft fabric measuring tape. Measure the following every two weeks:
- Chest
- Waist (at the smallest part)
- Hips (at the widest point, including your beautiful butt)
- Each thigh (at the thickest point)

To create and use your "test outfit," choose an outfit that fits you well right now and is not stretchy. It should be a pair of jeans or something with an unforgiving fabric. Put it away in a bag and label it "test outfit." In two weeks, try it on again to see if it is fitting any looser or tighter.

It is also helpful to take a photo of yourself. Modesty sucks, so get scantily clad and have someone you are comfy with take your photo. There is always a selfie option which most of us are terrible at taking. A profile, rear, and forward full-body shot are ideal. Keep those photos for reference of your before, during, and after weight-loss and fitness progress. Look at your photo and notice if your body composition visually changes.

We will discuss your exercise in detail when we move to the next chapter. Are you already exercising? Great! If you are not, document what is preventing you from exercise. Note mild and moderate exercise, including walking the baby. Document your exercise patterns in your journal, including time of day, type of exercise, and duration. Note how you are feeling. More energetic? Happier? Are your feelings of self-confidence and well-being improving? Regular exercise can increase your energy levels. It may seem counterintuitive, but research shows that expending energy by engaging in regular exercise will pay off with increased energy in the long run. The psychological benefits of regular physical activity include increased levels of self-esteem and better overall mood. When you exercise, your body releases chemicals called endorphins that give you a natural high and reduce stress. Note what type of exercise did you perform and for how long? If you skipped a planned fitness session, note why.

Sleeping patterns are very important to health and fitness. Every day, record the time you wake up and the time you go to bed so that you can be aware of your routine. Having a new baby is extremely disruptive to your sleep patterns.

It seems like as soon as you nod off to sleep, the baby wakes up hungry. This will get so much easier over time as baby sleeps for longer bouts. However, waking up mommy with bad dreams, loneliness, or illness will continue for many years. I found that after having my children, I became so hyper-aware that I now wake up at the sound of a pin drop. My seven-year-old still wakes me up to crawl into my bed, and I end up with his footie pajamas in my face. I wouldn't have it any other way; eventually they won't want to walk next to me at the shopping mall, so I will take the snuggles while I can have them. My mom-friends who have older children with driver's licenses also lack sleep waiting for their kids to come home safely. Once a mom, always a restless night.

Sleep is important because while you are sleeping, your body repairs damaged tissue, produces crucial hormones, and strengthens memory. Lack of sleep results in "Mommy C.R.S."—can't remember shit. Short stretches of sleep deprivation can be challenging but are not proven to have a long-term effect. However, lack of sleep can contribute negatively to the weight-loss effort. Too-little sleep boost the levels of hormones that make you feel hungry while reducing the secretion of hormones that make you feel full.

When people are sleep-deprived and eat a cookie, their blood sugar goes higher and they are more resistant to the effect of insulin than if they ate the same after a good night's sleep. Studies indicate that if you are on a diet to lose weight and you sleep less than five hours per night, 75 percent of the weight you will lose will be lean muscle mass. That indicates that just 25 percent of the weight you are losing is fat. Exercise is a great sleep aid. Exercising just before bedtime can make you less tired due to endorphins created during exercise. The best scenario is to exercise four or five hours prior to bedtime. Remember, when baby is little, ask your spouse to give a feeding so you can get a healthy stretch of sleep.

Now that you have begun your journal, review it at the end of the week. Read through your notes and discover the patterns that are challenging your progress. Things like being off schedule, conflicts at work, travel, hormones, and feeling overcommitted are just a few of the issues that can throw you off your fitness focus. Overeating can be the result of hormonal fluctuations or emotional stress. Be aware of your body chemistry and emotions. Understand and review your own documented words about why you eat, miss exercise, and miss sleep. Determining your challenges will enable you to overcome them! Identify the causes of these challenges in order to create solutions. Each week, write up a summary describing how much progress you have made toward your goals. This will be useful for long-term tracking and will help you identify patterns, such as why you are getting off track with your diet, exercise plan, or both.

# 6

# Something to Sweat About[5]

*Hollyism: "Smart women sweat."*

How soon after delivery of your baby can you realistically begin exercising? The American College of Obstetricians and Gynecologists (ACOG) says it's okay to gradually resume exercising as soon as you feel up to it. However, your doctor or midwife may want you to wait until your six-week postpartum checkup to advise you on exercise. If you have exercised throughout your pregnancy and had a normal vaginal delivery, you can safely do light exercise within days of giving birth. If you had a C-section, it may take at least several weeks to heal, resulting in a delay in resuming exercise. Even with a C-section, walking at a comfortable pace is advantageous because it promotes healing and helps prevent blood clots that can result from being sedentary.

If you are anything like me, you have likely been clothed in sweatpants for the first three months after birth. When I finally tried to get dressed in pre-pregnancy clothes,

---

[5] Video instruction on each exercise available. Visit YouTube: Holly Chisholm Hargrave, "Something to Sweat About."

I realized things had shifted. Inevitably, I caught a fleeting glimpse of myself in the mirror. Body dysmorphia! As a result of breastfeeding, total breast obliteration! Leaning over to dry my hair, I saw what used to be my voluptuous boobs reflected in the bathroom mirror. Now hanging like stretched goat tits, they swayed back and forth in the breeze of my hairdryer. All I thought was, "Who the hell is that in the mirror and what is my head doing on top of her body?" Off I went for my mammogram with my deflated balloons. The technician needed a spatula to peel the flattened flesh off of the machine. Time to move on to reconstructing your Hot Mommy body, and that requires muscle building. You might be thinking to yourself, "But my breasts are fat tissue." This is true. However, the pectoral muscles that support your breasts are among the strongest in your body. By strengthening the pectorals, you can regain definition and lift in your breast line. Only by building muscle can you actually change your body composition.

Wearing maternity clothes postpartum is perfectly normal. BabyCenter.com surveyed nearly 7,000 moms with babies ranging in age from just a few days old to four years old, and for most people, the weight loss was a struggle. Even the celebrities who lose the weight within three months have to work out regularly for extended amounts of time measured in hours, not minutes. This requires getting outside help with the baby and eating smart. It's hard work; there is no way around it. But you can do it. It is important to do it only when you are ready, not due to external pressure for perfection. A recent study indicated that 61 percent of new moms expected to be back down to their pre-pregnancy weight by their baby's first birthday. However, nearly 60 percent of all women were still carrying extra pounds. A year is a realistic timeline for a motivated new mom to lose her pregnancy weight. The key is to be motivated, dedicated, and smart by using the tools in this book. My belief is that it takes approximately a year to put the weight on and should take approximately the same to take the weight off.

The last ten pounds take the longest to shed; remain vigilant. Being busy and fatigued makes it hard to find time to exercise and eat right. In 2008, 37 percent of moms with two- to three-year-old children reported they were still holding on to ten or more pounds of their pregnancy weight. This year, that number has fallen to 22 percent.[6]

Are you ready to get back into your full-on fitness routine? If the answer is yes, then girls, get your sweat on. Join those moms with sexy physiques and glowing complexions. Exercise is the ultimate anti-aging product. Sweating from exercise keeps your pores clear and skin firm. Muscle mass fills in loose tummy and arm skin. Our skin loses elasticity as we age, causing that bra fat and crease under your butt cheeks. Muscle definition will help you to defy gravity and keep you looking young. Tone your triceps and biceps. When you wave goodbye, no hanging underarm dingle-dangle will echo your sentiments. The fabulous butt is my favorite muscle to keep lean and shredded up! The gluteus maximus is the biggest muscle in your body. Don't take that personally—it's the biggest muscle in everyone's body.

Keeping your glutes firm will help your butt look great, and the additional muscle mass will burn more calories

[6] Leslie Crawford and Sierra Senyak, "The New-Mom Body Survey: 7,000 Women Tell it Like it Is," *Baby Center*, n.d., http://www.babycenter.com/0_the-new-mom-body-survey-7-000-women-tell-it-like-it-is_3653252.bc

all day long. Importantly, women who exercise have greater longevity— both in the bedroom and in life—than those who don't. Women who exercise regularly enjoy stellar sex. Sex requires all sorts of muscle action. Increased endurance and a healthy body image from exercise allow you to maintain stamina and feel confident. Lights on, hot mom!

In the game of life, regular exercise has demonstrated a reduction in morbidity and mortality from many chronic diseases. Millions of Americans suffer from chronic illnesses that can be prevented or improved through regular physical activity. Don't be part of that statistic. Chronic diseases plague our nation. Fight back with fitness!

- 12.6 million people have coronary heart disease
- 1.1 million people suffer from a heart attack in a given year
- Seventeen million people have diabetes; about 90 to 95 percent of cases are type 2 diabetes, which is associated with obesity and physical inactivity
- Approximately sixteen million people have prediabetes
- 107 thousand people are diagnosed with colon cancer each year
- Three hundred thousand people suffer from hip fractures each year
- Fifty million people have high blood pressure[7]

Nearly fifty million adults between the ages of twenty and seventy-four—27 percent of the adult population—are obese. Overall, more than 108 million adults—61 percent of the adult population—are either obese or overweight. Nearly

[7] United States Department of Health and Human Services (DHHS), http://www.hhs.gov

80 percent of adults do not get the recommended amounts of exercise each week.[8] Are you sweating yet?

The U.S. government recommends adults get at least two-and-a-half hours of moderate-intensity aerobic exercise per week—such as brisk walking, one hour and fifteen minutes of vigorous-intensity activity, such as jogging or vigorous cycling—or a combination of the two. Adults should also engage in muscle-strengthening activities that work all the major muscle groups at least twice per week for thirty minutes, such as push-ups or weight lifting. As an alternative, you could do the same exercises for a shorter duration at a more vigorous level. An equivalent mix of moderate- and high-intensity aerobic activity can be combined to meet the total aerobic requirement of 150 minutes per week. [9]

I hear you; 150 minutes each week? How am I ever going to fit that into my schedule? You can break it up into smaller chunks of time during the day. If you need to break up your exercise into segments, target exercising at a moderate to vigorous effort for a minimum of ten minutes at a time.

---

[8] Centers for Disease Control and Prevention (CDC), http://www.cdc.gov

[9] Ryan Jaslow, "CDC: 80 Percent of American Adults Don't Get Recommended Exercise," CBS News, May 3, 2103, http://www.cbsnews.com/news/cdc-80-percent-of-american-adults-dont-get-recommended-exercise/

# 7

# Intimidation Factor

*Hollyism: "Balance is BEAUTIFUL. A healthy, balanced body equals a healthy, balanced life."*

Here is the elephant in the room—and I don't mean the post-pregnant mommy. Let me tell you how many clients I have had say to me, "I am going to come to your group class, but I have to get in shape first." What? That is the entire point of coming to class. So we said it: everyone is intimidated that somehow others are judging their appearance. Maybe we should make a T-shirt that says, "New Baby Momma" to wear to the gym. I actually got congratulated on my new pregnancy after I gave birth to my last baby. I wanted to cry!

In a too-big T-shirt and capris, I walked into the gym for what felt like was the first time in my life. I wondered why the hell the entire place had to be covered with full-length mirrors. Until then, I had enjoyed my waist-up mirror over my bathroom counter. The fluorescent lighting was way too bright, and I felt like they were spotlights on my cellulite thighs, flabby tummy, and fat butt. I felt like surely everyone was looking at me, and judging my body and readiness to exercise. Trust me girls, no one is looking at you. All those mirrors are there because every woman is looking at herself!

No one cares how you look; they only care how *they* look. Don't intimidate yourself by engaging in a self-deprecating mind game. My new client recently started exercising at my fitness studio and felt intimidated by others. Soon, she was approached by a woman asking her what she was doing to achieve her level of fitness. You might think of someone else's body as your "goal body," but it is likely that you are already someone else's "goal body." Congratulations! Life is not a competition, nor is exercise and fitness, unless you get your pro-competition card. If that is the case, remember me in your acknowledgments. You are the only one who matters today. You stuck with you and made it to the gym. It is your body and your time; forget everything else for this hour.

When engaging in exercise, be aware of yourself, mentally and physically. Awareness enables you to make better decisions. Being mentally present during exercise sessions is critical to proper form and injury prevention. I witness moms rushing into my fitness classes, throwing down their gym bags and jumping mindlessly into exercise. I clearly read that they are still not mentally in the present. They are just running through their to-do lists, worried about having time to get showered and to their next obligation.

During your exercise session, get out of the cerebral grocery line, the meeting, and the laundry. The ideal state of mind for action is awareness. Post-pregnancy, your joints are still loose, and balance can be compromised. Stay mentally present to prevent injury. If you feel pain—and you know the difference between sharp pain and the burn of exercise—back off your exertion. Now is the time to be kind to you.

# 8

# Effort Defines You

*Hollyism: "We can always make excuses, but we cannot make both excuses and PROGRESS."*

The best way to stick with fitness is to make a dedicated effort to find an exercise you enjoy. The key to dropping those pregnancy pounds is to do some form of exercise to get your heart rate pumping and your muscles toning. If you haven't exercised previously, or if in the past, you found exercise to be a chore, start by finding something you enjoy. Think about things in your life that you're most passionate about and make you feel your best. What activities do you find yourself gravitating toward? Do you envision yourself inside, outdoors, swimming, hiking, or pole dancing? Physical activity combined with healthy eating is the most effective way to lose weight. Let's get you moving in the right direction toward an activity that makes you smile. Explore different types of exercise programs and gather information about what you liked. Try new classes and a variety of sports. Explore ways to move your body that make you happy and do not cause you injury. Your fitness-oriented lifestyle must be sustainable, and fitness should be fun. Exercise variations are unlimited; search until you find what makes you look forward to exercise.

Sadly, many people associate exercise with punishment. A common thought process is, "We ate badly, so now we must exercise ninety minutes on the elliptical and take a spin class followed by seventy-five minutes of hot power yoga." Exercise bulimia is a real and serious disorder. Exercise bulimia is an eating disorder poised to become more threatening than anorexia or bulimia, and is characterized by excessive exercising, usually attached to feelings of guilt about eating. Millions of people in the United States suffer from diagnosed eating disorders—most of them women. This staggering statistic does not include the many women who remain silent.

Once you have established something you enjoy, literally book it on your calendar and do not skip your appointment. Always schedule your exercise session into your daily routine and respect it as you would a doctor's appointment. When something has to be dropped in your day, do not let it be your exercise session. I find if you can schedule exercise in the morning, it is best, due to the fact that the twists and turns of the day can impact your schedule. Whatever time of day your schedule permits, keep your exercise appointment as a priority. Join forces with a group or trainer to make you accountable to your exercise appointment. The Hot Mommy attitude is contagious. Grab a friend, hire a personal trainer, or find a group fitness class that you can attend regularly. A friend who shares your goals is great, and you can keep one another on track. A personal trainer is phenomenal! A qualified personal trainer can design a program to meet your specific fitness goals. Even better, when you have a commitment to your personal trainer, you will have an appointment you cannot skip.

Group classes are another great option. Things like yoga, spinning, and muscle sculpting group classes are available at your local fitness facility. The nice thing about group fitness classes is you will become part of a team of people who regularly attend that class. Knowing they are expecting to see you will keep you encouraged to participate. Accountability breeds success. We all deserve support. Don't hesitate to reach out and find your source. Join forces with positive energy people. Fitness is as contagious as a smile. If the gym is not for you, grab a friend from the neighborhood, look on a local town news website or local town flyers, search the Internet for a moms' fitness group in your city, or check the YMCA, local charity, or church organizations. There are many mommy/baby workout groups where you bring your baby along. Alternatively, other workout groups are available where new moms meet without their baby in tow. Bottom line, join a supportive mom team to keep yourself accountable and on track.

A support group of others who share your goals is instrumental to staying on track. This morning, in pouring rain and fifty-five-degree weather, I saw the most amazing sight: a group of walkers I typically see on my way to the fitness studio—rain coats on, hoods up, out for their daily exercise. I was inspired to see them and wondered if they didn't have one another to be accountable to, would they have walked alone on this cold, rainy morning? I noticed them laughing and saw the smiles on their faces. It was incredibly beautiful—truly a village of fitness girlfriends. We all deserve support.

Your body will ask a lot from you when you exercise, but your mind will ask much more. The ideal state of mind for action is awareness. Action creates energy, and energy use burns calories. When you are aware of your goals and potential pitfalls (such as being self-critical or not prioritizing your exercise), you gather more information regarding yourself and your circumstances. Mentally, the gift of being present during your exercise session is letting go of the mommy to-do list and enjoying the freedom and clarity of the moment. Focus on you, your body, your movements, and your purpose for being there, which we agree is to be the best you possible.

# 9

# Optimal Mommy Moves

*Hollyism: "Train how you want to look."*

What are the best overall exercises for new moms? A combination of cardiovascular and weight-bearing activity will obtain optimal results. If you want to hire a fitness trainer and need a test question to ensure they are qualified, ask them what the difference is between weight-bearing exercise and resistance-training exercise. If they don't know, don't hire them. The answer is simple. Weight-bearing exercise involves using your own body weight, as opposed to resistance training that requires external added weight via dumbbells and medicine balls.

As a new mom, weight-bearing exercise might be an ideal option when first starting, since there is no need for equipment or a gym. Don't be scared off from resistance training by the fear of bulking up. Can I tell you how many times I have had a new client ask me if weight training will bulk them up? I have to stop myself from replying, "Are you calling me a bulky she-man?" I curl sixty pounds with free weights, squat two hundred pounds with a barbell, and train six days a week. Trust me, you will not bulk up. The only way for us women to start growing a mustache and getting bulky is by producing more testosterone, taking steroids, or lifting extremely heavy weights. Being a bodybuilder takes specialized training and diet. Resistance training is key to sculpting your delicious body. You are going to lean out, your jeans will fit, and your ass will look tight. The only way to truly change your body shape is resistance training, not renewing your eyeglass prescription or getting liposuction.

Cardiovascular exercise is also referred to as cardio-respiratory. It involves movement that gets your heart rate up, which improves oxygen consumption by the body. Cardiovascular exercise helps you to lose weight and maintain weight loss. It also helps you build endurance so you can remain active for a longer period of time. This is critical in all facets of your life. The more energy you have, the more you can accomplish. Getting energy back post-pregnancy is critical to battle fatigue and achieve weight loss. Begin by walking briskly with your baby in a jogging stroller, then progress to a light run, catch your breath by slowing to a walk, then progress to a jog again. Work your way up to jogging for thirty minutes.

If you can't get to a gym and weather doesn't permit, consider investing in a treadmill or other piece of cardio equipment like a stationary bike for your home. Many are made to be space-friendly. With my last baby, Hudson, I opted to buy a treadmill for my home. I was beyond tired and didn't want to lug three babies to childcare at a gym. I began by walking briskly on my treadmill, my heart pounding in utter misery under my added pounds of baby fat. I progressed to a light jog and felt every pound I was carrying.

Everything, my friends, becomes mental at this stage of the health and fitness game. Focusing on maintaining my effort, I kept a watchful eye on Hudson. He safely sat and watched cartoons while drooling on a large play ball in his adorable footie pajamas. You will hit obstacles; we all do. There will be pitfalls. Focus on moving forward, not looking back. Where there is a will, there is a way.

## HOLLY'S TOP 7 BACK AND ABDOMINAL WEIGHT-BEARING EXERCISES

**1** "SUPERMOMS"

- Back strengthening
- Equipment: none

In the initial days, it is hard to find baby-free time, so have fun by engaging in creative exercises with your baby. This is an exercise you can do while watching your baby. Lay your baby on a blanket on the floor in front of you. You lay on your tummy facing your baby. Begin with your forehead, arms, and legs on the floor. Now, lift your face for a game of "peek-a-boo" and look at your baby laugh. As you perform this, also lift your arms and feet off the floor. This movement is called a "superman," but let's call it a "supermom." Lift fifteen times. Rest and repeat three sets of fifteen.

When you can carve out some baby-free time, the following are my recommendations based on effectiveness and efficiency. These exercises work both your abdominals and back simultaneously.

## 2   "POINTERS"

- Back Strengthening
- Equipment: none

This exercise can be performed while watching your baby or on your own. If with baby, lay your baby on a blanket on the floor in front of you. Position yourself on hands and knees (tabletop position). Lift your opposite hand and leg simultaneous while looking forward at your baby. Lift your right hand to shoulder level and pretend you are reaching toward your baby or the wall in front of you. Lift your left foot to back level and envision kicking the wall behind you. Engage your abdominals as if you are lifting them off the fabric of your shirt. Return to resting position on hands and knees. Repeat fifteen times on each side—right hand/left leg then left hand/right leg. Repeat for three sets of fifteen on each side.

## 3   "PLANK HOLD"

- Abdominal and back strengthening
- Equipment: none

A plank is holding your body strong like a board on your hands and feet with your body lifted to arm level, back straight, and glutes in line with your back. You can begin on your elbows if being on your arms is initially too straining. Hold a plank for as long as possible and repeat three times. Time your progress with a clock, cell phone, or other device. Try and start with a fifteen-second hold, progress to thir-ty-seconds, and finally progress to a one-minute hold. Rest and repeat the hold for three sets.

# 4   "SUSPENDED PLANK ON BODY BALANCE BALL"

- Abdominal and back strengthening
- Equipment: body balance ball. A body ball is a large, inflatable ball you can purchase in different diameters. It comes flattened in a box with a hand pump.

Hold a plank position with a body ball under your ankles and your legs out straight. In order to get into this position, roll yourself over the body ball until it is beneath your ankles, then lift onto your arms so that you are in a suspended plank position. The body ball will make your balance much more challenging. Hold a plank for as long as possible. Time your progress with a clock, cell phone, or other device. Try and start with a fifteen-second hold, progress to thirty-seconds, and finally progress to a one-minute hold. Rest and repeat the hold for three sets. You may fall off the ball now and again—we all do. A sense of humor is required to be a mother, so it's good practice to laugh at yourself.

# 5   "SUSPENDED PLANK ON BODY BALANCE BALL WITH ABS CRUNCH"

- Abdominal and back strengthening
- Equipment: body balance ball

Hold a plank position with a body ball under your ankles and your legs out straight. In order to get into this position, roll yourself over the body ball until it is beneath your ankles, then lift onto your arms so that you are in a suspended plank position. Utilizing your abdominals, crunch your knees into your chest and return to a perfect plank position. Repeat fifteen repetitions of crunching knees to chest to plank. On the fifteenth repetition, hold your body in a plank position and count to ten. Rest and repeat for three sets of fifteen with the ten-count hold.

### 6 "PASS THE BODY BALANCE BALL"

- Abdominal strengthening
- Equipment: body balance ball

Lie on your back and place the body ball between your feet on the floor with legs fully extended and a slight break in the knee. Your hands are on the floor above your head. Pressing your abdominals into your spine and your spine into the floor, reach your arms up while lifting the ball to your arms with your legs. Pass the body ball from your feet to your hands with a full extension between movements. When the ball is between your feet and your feet are on the floor, your arms are on the floor above your head. Pass the ball so it is now in your hands above your head and your feet are on the floor. Muscle is built on the extension; full extension is critical to maximum results. Repeat for fifteen repetitions. Rest and repeat for three sets of fifteen.

### 7 "BODY BALANCE BALL ROLLOUT"

Abdominal and back strengthening
Equipment: body balance ball

Kneel down in front of the body ball. Interlock your fingers and place them at the halfway point of the top of the ball and the floor. Roll your body out while rolling the ball forward until you are in a perfect plank. Next, use your abdominals, pressing your belly button into your spine, to roll the ball back into the starting position. Repeat for fifteen repetitions. Rest and repeat for three sets of fifteen.

Once you regain your basic strength, it is important to add resistance training to your routine. Resistance training is defined as the use of weights or resistance bands in order to gain muscle mass. The more muscle you gain, the more strength you will have to manage your baby and the more calories you will burn. Muscle burns up to fifty more calories per pound per day than fat does. Increasing muscle increases your metabolism—the rate at which you burn calories. Transferring five pounds of fat to five pounds of muscle can potentially burn an additional 250 calories per day! That is 1,750 calories burned per week, excluding cardiovascular exercise. I recommend the following back and abdominal exercises using weights to increase muscle strength.

## HOLLY'S TOP 7 BACK AND ABDOMINAL RESISTANCE TRAINING EXERCISES: LEVEL ADVANCED

### 1 "WEIGHTED SIDE PLANK"

- Back and abdominal strengthening
- Equipment: three- to five-pound free weights/ dumbbells

Assume a slide plank position. Perform this by rolling on your side, stacking your feet, and lifting your body on one arm. Holding one weight in your free hand, raise the weight to the ceiling and follow your hand holding the weight with your eyes. With control, lower the weight and place it through the bottom of your waist between your body and the floor as you hold your back and abdominals strong in the side plank position. Repeat fifteen times on your right side and fifteen times on your left side. Rest and repeat three times. If holding the full side plank is initially too challenging, rest on your elbow.

## 2 "ADVANCED WEIGHTED POINTERS"

- Back and abdominal strengthening
- Equipment: set of two free weights, three or five pounds

Get on the floor on your hands and knees. Hold one weight under each hand. Lift the weight to shoulder height with a straight elbow. Simultaneously, lift your opposite leg and kick it out at back height to the wall behind you. Your right hand with the weight is lifted straight forward to shoulder level while your left foot is lifted to back level kicking the wall behind you. Engage your abdominals as if you are lifting them off the fabric of your shirt. Next, pull your arm in and, using your abdominals, reverse crunch the weight to your opposite knee, pulling the knee and the arm together until the weight touches the knee. Now, fully extend the arm and leg and repeat for fifteen repetitions on the same arm and leg. Do not return to resting position on hands and knees until the repetitions are complete. Repeat fifteen times on each side, (right hand/ left leg, then left hand/right leg). Repeat for three sets of fifteen on each side.

### 3  "WEIGHTED SUPER MOMS"

- Back strengthening
- Equipment: five-pound dumbbell

Lay on the floor on your stomach. Hold one dumbbell by each end in both of your hands. Raise your arms, lifting the dumbbell as high as you can while simultaneously lifting both of your legs off the floor. Lift fifteen times. On the fifteenth repetition, hold the position fully engaged with the dumbbell and legs raised and count to ten, remembering to breathe. Rest and repeat three sets of fifteen.

### 4  "BODY BALANCE BALL REVERSE FLIES"

- Back strengthening
- Equipment: body balance ball and set of dumbbells, three or five pounds

Lay over the body balance ball on your stomach with your chest just over the balance ball and your feet on the ground. Take one weight in each hand. Lift your upper body as high as you can and engage your back and glutes. Perform a reverse fly on the ball. A reverse fly is opening your arms like a bird opening its wings to take off for flight. Pull your shoulders together on the opening like you are trying to grasp a pencil between your shoulder blades. Repeat fifteen repetitions. Rest and repeat for three sets.

## 5  "WEIGHTED ABDOMINAL CRUNCHES"

- Abdominal strengthening
- Equipment: three- or five-pound free weight

Holding one free weight in both hands, extend your arms above your head while lying on your back. Perform a classic crunch, tapping the weight to your toes. Do this by pushing your abdominals into your spine and your spine into the floor. Extend your legs fully to the floor and return your arms to start position on the floor above your head. Repeat fifteen repetitions. Rest and repeat for three sets.

## 6  "WEIGHTED ABDOMINAL REVERSE PIKE"

- Abdominal strengthening
- Equipment: three- or five-pound free weights

Hold one free weight in each hand while lying flat on the floor with your arms extended above your head. Raise your legs straight up with little to no break in the knees, and raise your upper body to touch the weights to your feet. Your body will resemble the letter "V." Tap the weights to your toes and return to the start position. If this is too challenging initially, you can begin by holding one weight in both hands.

## 7  "WEIGHTED SEATED OBLIQUE"

- Abdominal strengthening
- Equipment: Three- or five-pound free weight

Begin in a sitting position with your heels down on the floor and your toes pointed up to the ceiling. Lean back, engaging your abs and back. Keep your back straight. If it begins to strain, decrease the level at which you are leaning back. You can also place a ball below your lower back for support as needed. This seated, leaning back position is called "boat pose." If you have the strength, you can lift your feet to hover just above the floor. Holding one weight in both hands, tap it as far as you can behind you to your left and then to your right. Twist through your side abdominals while keeping your hips in line with your feet. The movement is focused through your waist. Follow the weight with your eyes. Keeping your eyes on the weight increases your range of motion up to 30 percent, which increases your muscle progress and range of motion. Tap left and right thirty times, which equals a full set (left and right) of fifteen repetitions. Rest and repeat three times.

# 10

# The Skinny on Sex

*Hollyism: "Lights on, hot mom."*

The truth about sex after childbirth is that it's not the same; at least not right away. Things were going along just fine in the sex department until around nine months later, when out popped a wailing newborn. Body changes, family changes, and new responsibilities make post-baby sex challenging.

Your sex drive typically revs back up around six weeks after giving birth, but can sometimes take up to—sorry to say—between six months and one year. Your body image might make you shy away from sex. Let that one go, ladies. Don't dwell on how your body has changed; you are sexy. Your vagina, however, might not feel the same way.

It is something none of us really want to hear, but after childbirth, many women have looser vaginas. Health experts say the best thing women can do, post-delivery, is Kegel exercises, which can help tighten your vaginal and pelvic floor muscles. These mimic trying to hold your pee in traffic. Even if you had a normal birth experience with minimal trauma, you can expect a bit of pain the first time you have sex again. If you had vaginal tears—yipes! I had three C-sections; oh, the burning reminder of those stitches feeling like they were ripping out with sex—ouch! If you are breastfeeding, it is normal for moms to feel like, "Everyone step away from my milk-squirting boobs and burning va-jay-jay!" Am I scaring you? Nah, this is super temporary! It too shall pass; I'm just assuring you that it's normal, my friends. We all go through it, and it's okay; you are more desirable than ever.

When you are ready, sex is just as delicious in the post-children phase of life as in pre-children. You just have to work a little harder to—excuse my pun—fit it in. Girls, our sexual prime is thriving during our thirties, and women in their forties report having the best sex of their lives. My solution to the challenge of finding time for sex after having children is to put a lock on your bedroom door. Convinced the baby is napping or your older children are otherwise distracted, you quickly lock the door for sex. In the building heat and breaking sweat, you predictably hear, "Mommy, I need you!" Mommy's natural response is to tell hubby to hurry up and satisfy himself. Are we nuts? Hurry up? Don't we deserve an orgasm? Turn up the volume on the music so you can't hear the kids yelling for you for something silly like changing the television channel. Unless they are screaming fire, ignore them. I am not saying for hours. I am saying give yourself five minutes. Assuming, of course, you have left them in a super-safe environment—which you have, because you're Supermom.

Don't wait until bedtime when you are too exhausted to enjoy sex. Sneaking naughty, hot sex is arousing. Your kids have no idea what you are doing, so drop the paranoia. If they are old enough to know what you are up to, then you need to get past it. Look, your kids are going to end up in therapy over your parenting for something, so choose your battles.

Sex positions work a multitude of muscle groups. Powerful sex can substitute for a workout session at the gym. Tighten your glutes, engage your thighs, and SEXERCISE. Abdominals shift into your ribcage as you engage your lover. Use your biceps to tighten your grip on his back and ass. Your strong arms will pull him deep inside you. Tighten your lower back in a pelvic tilt for ultimate penetration. Sweat!

Countless studies indicate the benefits of sex for your mental and physical health. Sex burns calories and releases endorphins and other feel-good hormones. These hormones powerfully affect our feelings of satisfaction and reward. Goodbye fat-holding stress, hello calorie-burning, hot sex! Interestingly enough, a reduction in stress also increases your sexual desire; the more sex you have, the more sex you crave. An object in motion remains in motion—calories out!

Sex is more satisfying when you exercise regularly. Don't you deserve an orgasm or three? Turn up the sexual fire by tuning up your physical fitness. Countless studies indicate the benefits of physical health to maximize sexual satisfaction. Exercise burns calories, increases blood flow to the genitals, and releases feel-good hormones. Wild sex has the same physical and psychological effects as exercise. Imagine the ultimate climax when your exercise and sex coincide!

A fit body fosters a greater sense of self-confidence. Self-esteem is critical to sizzling sex. You need not achieve the "perfect body" to be confident. Self-assurance provided by regular exercise will beguile your sense of sexual desire and physical allurement. Be self-aroused by knowing you are sexually exciting—lights on and mirrors!

Let's review the best exercises to improve your Hot Mommy sex life, starting with cardiovascular exercise. Increased stamina via high-intensity interval training adds a spark to your sex life. If you're out of cardiovascular shape, you are likely doing disservice to your sex life. High-intensity interval training will give you a cardiovascular—as in heart-racing—boost in the bedroom. Things like running, indoor cycling or spinning, using an elliptical, and swimming will do the trick. Target thirty to forty minutes of your best effort.

Strength training is also great for better sex—things like a weighted Pilates squat. The weighted Pilates squat is an ultimate strength exercise to improve your intimacy in the bedroom. Strong gluteus muscles enable you to balance yourself in multiple positions. A tight gluteus not only looks attractive, it is a main center of balance in the body. Inner and outer thigh tone is sexy to gaze upon and provides the ability to squeeze your partner nice and tightly. The ability to open your hips is beneficial in many sexual ways by helping you and your lover enjoy flexibility while molding your bodies together in a comfortable intimate position.

Yoga and flexibility training is also helpful for playtime in the bedroom. Upward dog is a yoga pose that will enable you to strengthen your arms, shoulders, quads, thighs, and core muscles, as well as elongate your abdominal wall. This pose is multi-functional. Full-body muscle strength will enable you to confidently hold a strong and sexy position over your lover.

Try yoga or Pilates to flex your limbs into creative arrangements and seriously up the fun factor in bed. Strength is key, but flexibility really pays off when it comes to creativity. Flexibility allows you to be adventurous when it comes to trying new sex positions. The "Happy Baby" position will open up your inner thighs when you are on top or below your partner. The ability to open your thighs is important in preventing leg cramps. It also aids in your ability to relax your legs while opening your thighs, enhancing the comfort and therefore the sexual encounter. To perform "Happy Baby," lie on your back and hold your feet with your hands inside your legs. Rock your body gently back and forth and side to side like a happy baby.

Research has not determined precisely how long sex lasts on average. A normal time could be anywhere from two minutes (a quickie for who?) to an hour or more if you have the time for foreplay and after play. Women prefer external stimulation. If the kids are making you crazy, send your husband out of the bedroom to manage them, and allow yourself some private sexuality. Grab your favorite toy and orgasm yourself! Happy mommy equals happy family.

The number of calories you burn during sex depends on your weight, the duration of sex, and your vigor. Show enthusiasm. An average, 150-pound person will burn 216 calories in a forty-five-minute session. Foreplay also burns calories, so make foreplay last as long as possible! Keep your heart rate up and your blood pumping with lots of playtime. Make sex last longer by chilling out the pace. It is not a sprint. Experiment with different positions, kissing, and massage. Be creative!

A tip for your man: men who masturbate a few hours prior to sex prolong ejaculation in the next experience. Reaching orgasm can burn an additional sixty to one hundred calories. Multiple orgasms? Do the math! The secret to burning calories during sex is turning up the passion.

## BURNING UP CALORIES IN THE SHEETS: A SUMMARY OF SEX SIZZLERS (BASED ON A 150-POUND INDIVIDUAL)

**1 PASSIONATE KISSING: SIXTY-EIGHT CALORIES PER HOUR**

Add a little petting and you approach ninety calories per hour. Make kissing and petting playful and erotic. Get your blood pumping with excitement and anticipation. Jai-ya Kinzbach, a Los Angeles–based sexologist and the author of *Red Hot Touch*, recommends kissing in unusual positions. She advises planking over your mate and kissing in a push-up position. Push-ups burn 171 calories in thirty minutes.

**2 SENSUAL UNDRESSING OF YOUR PARTNER: EIGHT OR MORE CALORIES**

The act of taking clothes off burns around eight to ten calories. An Italian researcher reportedly found that a man attempting to remove a bra with his mouth burned as many as eighty calories. Add a little sexy striptease to turn yourself on while turning on your partner and turning up the calorie-burning heat!

### 3   SEXUAL INTERCOURSE: FROM TWO HUNDRED CALORIES PER FORTY-FIVE MINUTES OR MORE

The key is duration and energy; make it hot and make it last. Engage your thighs and glutes, and move your hips. Release your inhibitions. Keep the lights on, love your body, and feel your self-esteem glow!

### 4   GIVING ORAL SEX: ONE HUNDRED CALORIES PER HALF-HOUR

Be generous; the giving end of oral sex may be just as effective as a quick sprint. Again, play with positions. A little yoga can increase your flexibility and fat burning.

Use sexy, healthy foods to turn up the heat in your love life. Aphrodisiacs were first sought out as a remedy for various sexual anxieties including fear of inadequate performance. There are lots of cliché foods like oysters and those with phallic shapes, but beyond that, there exist some simple, healthy alternatives.

According to researchers, the best things to eat for your sex life are those that are also best for your heart health. Clogged arteries impair circulation and the required blood flow to your body parts needed for satisfying sex. Oatmeal with flaxseed and raisins lowers cholesterol and indirectly increases blood vessel dilation. Blood vessel dilation is critical for strong blood flow. Salmon provides essential fatty acids that improve circulation by clearing cholesterol. Therefore, salmon helps to improve your blood flow. The omega-3s in salmon assist in hormone function and may increase feel-good hormone levels in your brain to add to your sexual arousal. Blueberries are yet another potential arouser. Soluble fiber in blueberries combats cholesterol to support healthy blood flow. Everyone agrees chocolate makes you feel in love. That is because chocolate contains phenyl ethylamine, which is a stimulant, and tryptophan, a brain chemical involved in sexual arousal.[10]

Examples of healthy aphrodisiac foods:

- Almonds
- Asparagus
- Avocado
- Garlic
- Ginger
- Oysters

---

[10] Corrie Pikul, "4 Foods That Can Improve Your Sex Life," *TheHuffingtonPost.com*, September 18, 2013, http://www.huffingtonpost.com/2013/09/18/best-foods-for-sex_n_3915457.html?utm_hp_ref=own-healthy

# 11

# Dieting Sucks

*Hollyism: "Eating is Nutrition, not Recreation."*

Diet is a four-letter word. Put a quarter in a jar for every time you use it! When I use the word "diet," I am referring to fad and/or crash dieting. These diets are based on severely restricted eating. Most fad diets require people to make drastic changes in their eating such as strictly limiting certain foods. For example, some diets suggest no sugar or carbohydrates, while others suggest very high protein or fat intake. Most fad diets are risky, and some are dangerous.

Most people simply cannot sustain a restrictive diet that is not congruent with their lifestyle. Simply stated, one style does not fit all. It's a fact: quick-fix, fad diets do not work long-term. There is no quick fix to weight loss. Only 5 percent of people who lose weight on a fad or crash diet will keep the weight off.[11] According to Dr. Gary Foster, clinical director of The Weight and Eating Disorders Program at the University of Pennsylvania, an average of 65 percent of fad dieters return to their pre-dieting weight within three years.

[11] Alex O'Meara, "The Percentage of People Who Regain Weight after Rapid Weight Loss and the Risks of Doing So," *Livestrong.com*, February 18, 2015, http://www.livestrong.com/article/438395-the-percentage-of-people-who-regain-weight-after-rapid-weight-loss-risks/

Healthy weight loss that lasts a lifetime requires a balanced approach and a long-term commitment. When approaching your weight loss via eating, think of it as a lifestyle change that is congruent with your family, your schedule, and your lifestyle.

During my last pregnancy, I gained fifty pounds. Convinced the boxes of Vienna finger cookies I consumed were validated, I ate them by the case—not to mention the endless amount of munchkins I devoured. I have asked many of my mommy clients how many munchkins they think equal a donut. There is never a hesitation; the answer is consistently a solid number five.

Cravings during pregnancy are common, due to fluctuating hormones and fatigue. My son, Hudson, weighed seven pounds at birth. In spite of my diligent exercise during my pregnancy, my eating was so beyond bad, that I packed on some serious pounds. Enter reality: Hudson was now out of my belly and I still had forty-five pounds left to lose. Forty-five pounds…YIPES! Trust me, I spent my days in pajamas or sweatpants for months. It is okay, it really is; you will prevail and regain fitting into your favorite blue jeans with time, patience, and dedication.

Weight loss and maintenance requires eating strategically. It does not mean starving yourself on some fad you can't maintain for a lifetime. Rewire your mentality about food. Eating is to fuel your body. Be aware of "why" you eat. Your journal will aid in deciphering your eating habits. Be sure to review your notes to educate yourself on why you ate at any given time. Eating out of stress, boredom, or—my personal favorite—"recreational eating," will kill your efforts to lose weight. By reviewing your journal weekly, you will become aware of why and when you eat. Remember to review your daily journal to understand your eating patterns.

We are all wired to eat for different emotional and physical reasons. Coming from a primarily Italian family, food for me represents love. Growing up, we ate when we were happy, sad, on holidays…hunger didn't matter. I remember my grandmother saying, "You need to finish your pasta," as she added an additional pile to my plate, "in order to have dessert." When I was full of pasta to the point of virtual explosion, I recall her saying, "You don't need to be hungry to eat dessert." Understand, she lived through the Great Depression and her heart was unquestionable. The point of the story is we all have our personal relationship with food. As an adult, you now have an ingrained relationship with food. Be aware of what food represents for you. For example, if food represents reward, reward yourself with a new piece of clothing, a massage, pedicure, or facial. Better yet, take the time to sit down and read this book.

Three meals a day went out with film cameras and DVD players. We are not only going to update what foods you eat, but we are going to change how you eat. Planning is critical, both when you eat—time and frequency—and what you eat—nutritional quality and source of calories.

Beginning with breakfast, target five small meals a day. Eating approximately every three hours should be your goal. Did you ever notice those people who seem to be eating healthy snacks constantly tend to be thin? That is because they are fueling their body and their metabolism. Frequent eating of smaller meals keeps your metabolic rate burning. It also shrinks the size of your stomach so you get full faster. Be a grazer. If you eat a little something when you are hungry, you are less likely to overeat later. It is better to taper calories during the day, than increasing them. Dinner should be your smallest meal of the day. Your 1,500-calorie-day should look something like this:

- 6:00 a.m. – breakfast: 350 calories
- 10:00 a.m. – snack: 250 calories
- 1:00 p.m. – lunch: 350 calories
- 4:00 p.m. – snack: 250 calories
- 7:00 p.m. – dinner: 300 calories

Eating this way helps you stay off the blood sugar roller coaster. Think about how easy it is to get off track in balanced eating. In the morning rush, you skipped breakfast or only had coffee. Late morning, your blood sugar has plummeted. Now you feel tired, cranky, and moody. Via two donuts and more coffee, you salvage yourself, and your blood sugar levels spike. Due to the late morning madness snacking, you decide to skip lunch and save calories. Busy with work, chores, or errands, you start to get foggy brain syndrome because now your blood sugar has dropped. The late afternoon lull is where the dreaded recovery eating begins—cookies, candy bar, and potato chips. You are seeking rapid energy and any sugar or simple carbohydrate will satiate you. Another sugar spike! By dinnertime, you aren't hungry. You crash—hard—and eat a too-big, late night meal. Curb your crazy by eating frequent, healthy meals to maintain your blood sugar levels at a steady, happy state.

# 12

# Nutri-Mom

*Hollyism: "Be smart to your body."*

Making good choices requires you to be informed of basic nutrition. This information will help you be a better eater for yourself and a better educator for your children. Let's begin with defining fuel sources and how they represent energy for your beautiful body.

Calories represent units of energy:

- Carbohydrates consist of four calories per gram
- Proteins consist of four calories per gram
- Fats consist of nine calories per gram
- Alcohols consist of seven calories per gram— almost as calorically dense as fat!

Carbohydrates are a primary fuel source for activity. When choosing a carbohydrate, avoid refined carbs. I like to refer to these carbs as "on your thighs carbs." They are seductive things like candy bars and white pasta. You can either wear Italian designer clothes or eat Italian food. You cannot do both. Generally, carbs should be sought from nutrient-dense, complex carb foods such as vegetables, fruits, and unprocessed grains. Complex carbohydrates contain the vitamins and minerals necessary to efficiently convert to gradual-release energy and will not cause a spike in your blood sugar level, as will refined carbs. When we are tired, we tend to go for those refined carbs and enjoy that almost instantaneous high state of energy, often followed by a crash and burn. This can lead to erratic eating patterns and will sabotage your goal to eat healthy.

Protein will increase your metabolism. Starting at age thirty, most people begin to lose around a half-pound of muscle each year. That muscle is necessary to turn up the Hot Mommy calorie-burning heat. Protein is not a main source of energy like carbohydrates and fat. Rather, it plays an important role in providing amino acids for your body. Protein becomes a critical source of energy when carbohydrate intake is too low. It supports muscle, bone, organ, tendon, and ligament strength. It is also critical in forming enzymes and hormones that send messages through the body's bloodstream for the thyroid, adrenal glands, the pancreas, and other organs to function properly. Protein also aids in blood transport and blood clotting and is essential for daily tissue maintenance and repairing and maintaining the fluid balance inside and outside cells.

Protein supports weight loss. It is low in calories, slows digestion, boosts metabolism, and promotes water loss. Protein can make you feel full longer. The recommended daily allowance (RDA) of protein for non-exercising individuals is 0.8 grams per kilogram of body weight. Unlike fat or carbohydrates, protein cannot be stored. For that reason, it is recommended to target 1.5 grams per kilogram of body weight. This is so that you feed the muscle you are building via your workouts.

Food intake changes will be in both quality and quantity of the foods you eat. While you are becoming accustomed to serving sizes, measure your food. Purchase a food scale, a two-cup measuring cup, and a six-cup measuring cup. Start measuring out your portions so you become visually familiar with appropriate serving sizes.

## GUIDE TO SERVING SIZES:

- Chicken, lean beef, and fish: three ounces (about the size of the palm of your hand)
- Egg whites: five whites
- Yam: 1 medium yam
- Vegetables: 1 cup
- Leafy greens: four cups
- Non-fat Greek yogurt: one cup
- No salt added cottage cheese: one-half cup
- Berries: one-half cup
- Apple: one medium apple
- Banana: one medium banana
- Almonds: one-quarter cup
- Grains: one-quarter cup
- Legumes/beans: one-quarter cup

To read a nutritional label, begin with the serving information at the top of the label. This will tell you the serving size of a single serving and the total number of servings per container.

Next, check total calories per serving size. This is important because the calories per serving and how many servings you're actually consuming add up to more calories than you might think if you eat the entire package. For example, if you double the servings you eat, you double the amount of calories.

The next section of information on a nutrition label shows the amounts of specific nutrients in the food. The American Heart Association (AHA) recommends you limit certain nutrients. Based on a two thousand calorie per day diet, AHA recommends no more than eleven to thirteen grams of saturated fat, as little trans-fat as possible, and no more than fifteen hundred milligrams of sodium. Their guidelines recommend to be sure you get enough of beneficial nutrients such as: dietary fiber, protein, calcium, iron, vitamins, and other nutrients you need every day. The percent of Daily Value (DV) tells you the percentage of each nutrient in a single serving. In review of the daily-recommended amount versus your personal nutritional goals use the following as a guide. If you want to consume less of a nutrient (such as saturated fat or sodium), choose foods with a lower percentage of DV—five percent or less. If you want to consume more of a nutrient (such as fiber), seek foods with a higher percentage of DV—twenty percent or more.[12]

---

[12] "Understanding Food Nutrition Labels," *American Heart Association*, October, 2014, http://www.heart.org/HEARTORG/GettingHealthy/NutritionCenter/HealthyEating/Understanding-Food-Nutrition-Labels_UCM_300132_Article.jsp

# 13

# A.O.B.—Alcohol on Board

*Hollyism: "Everything looks better with alcohol except the next morning."*

Drinking wine while preparing dinner can be relaxing. However, it can result in overeating. I call it "A.O.B.," meaning Alcohol On Board, and I recommend you don't drink and dine. Good decisions are seldom made with alcohol on board! Your tattoo might not be there if you hadn't been out drinking tequila with the girls! Alcohol makes you more likely to dance on the bar and have mind-blowing sex. The only bad thing is if you fall off the bar, the fab sex is with a stranger (in which case, see your OB/GYN as soon as possible), and alcohol makes you fat.

One glass of wine is around 110 calories. A glass a day quickly adds up to 770 calories per week. Alcohol and weight loss are enemies. Alcohol increases appetite, adds empty calories, and alters the digestive process. An occasional drink has its place in a healthy lifestyle. In fact, evidence shows that one glass of wine per day can reduce blood pressure, and red wine, in particular, has been noted to be heart-healthy. Alcohol is calorically dense, at seven calories per gram—almost as much as fat—and offers no nutritional value. Let's admit, it is hard to have just one drink.

Can you drink and lose weight? Yes, but it's inviting another challenge. Cocktails on ladies' night out, beer at the bar, wine with dinner; most of us enjoy a drink (or two or three) every now and again. Simply, alcohol can sabotage your weight-loss efforts.

If you're serious about losing weight, it's best to put alcohol aside until you're in maintenance mode. If you are going to have a drink, choose wine, which may protect the heart and help lower inflammation. You could also choose a drink with clear alcohol and no sugary mixers, such as vodka and club soda or tequila on the rocks with lime. One drink a day probably maxes out the benefits, though, so keep a cork in your alcohol consumption.

Alcohol is viewed as a toxin by your body. On an empty stomach, alcohol quickly goes to your head. As alcohol reaches the liver for processing, the liver places all of its attention on ridding it from our body. When the body is focused on processing alcohol, it is unable to properly break down foods containing carbohydrates and fat. These calories are then converted into unwanted fat stores in your body. YUCK.

Alcohol is a diuretic and causes dehydration. Do you ever wake up in a desert of thirst after an evening of drinking? With the water loss, you also lose important minerals including magnesium, potassium, calcium, and zinc. These minerals are vital to good health. It will put you to sleep, but will inhibit you from sleeping properly, causing you to awaken feeling tired. The resulting fatigue can trigger you to overeat the following day in search of an energy boost.

Both wine and beer contain carbohydrates and calories. Alcoholic beverages only have a few calories less than beer or wine. Avoid drinks that are boosted with sugar-laden fruit juices, which are just more added calories. An average cocktail contains around one hundred calories per shot. If you are going to add something to it, consider adding a squeeze of fresh lime and a spritz of seltzer. The sweeter the drink, the more calories it has. Dry wines usually have fewer calories than sweet cocktails and wines.

## ALCOHOL CALORIE GUIDE[13]

| Alcohol | Serving Size | Calories | Carbs |
|---|---|---|---|
| White Wine | 5 ounces | 110 | 4 |
| Red Wine | 5 ounces | 110 | 1 |
| Champagne | 4 ounces | 85 | 2 |
| Vodka | 2 ounces | 135 | 0 |
| Tequila | 2 ounces | 135 | 0 |
| Beer (Amstel Light) | 12 ounces | 100 | 5 |
| Cosmopolitan | 1 med. drink | 215 | 12 |
| Margarita | 1 med. drink | 160 | 7 |
| Pina Colada (10g. fat) | 1 med. drink | 325 | 26 |
| Long Island Iced Tea | 1 med. drink | 270 | 32 |

[13] Allan Borushek, *The CalorieKing: Calorie, Fat, & Carbohydrate Counter*, 1st ed. (Costa Mesa, CA: Family Health Publications, 2009).

Don't panic; you can have a drink or even a night of drinking and you won't burst into caloric flames. The key is moderation. Initially, try not to drink during the week. Sometimes, it is more the ceremony of a cocktail that helps you feel chill. Put your non-alcoholic beverage in a wine glass if that helps you to relax. If you feel like you can't avoid drinking, eat a healthy meal first. You will find that when you are full, you will not want to drink alcohol. If you are planning to have a night out, add an extra thirty minutes of exercise to balance your caloric intake.

Another little secret: order a vodka, tequila, or scotch on the rocks, and order a glass of water. As you sip—and I insist, sip—your cocktail, slyly add a bit of your ice water to your cocktail glass. You will find that one cocktail lasting you an evening that you might normally have had three, and triple the calories. Shh, our secret. Another choice when out imbibing is to have one glass of water between each glass of alcohol. At home, during the witching hour (dinner time), if you find yourself terrifying your family with a wicked bitch temper because you want that glass of wine, have just one and chill out. It's better than your best friend at your door because you drank the entire bottle in a tizzy of crazed stress. Ding-dong...I love you...pajamas...bedtime...night-night.

# 14

# Disaster Detours

*Hollyism: "Your past is not your potential. Avoid being your own worst critic. Yesterday was an experience; today is what you make it."*

It takes an average of twenty minutes for your mind to register that your stomach is full. Slow down and give yourself time to eat and recognize being full. My Hot Mommy Secret is to make my plate, then split it in half and put half away in the fridge. I eat the half on my plate, and I wait. Nine times out of ten, I don't need the other half.

Do a little science experiment for yourself. Each day you are disciplined enough to not clear your plate, rather than putting the leftovers in the trash, put them in a container in the fridge. Do this for one week. Throw your scraps in the same container and watch them pile up. At the end of one week, look inside of your container to see the uneaten food piled up. You will be amazed at how much food—and thereby, calories—you would have packed on if you had taken those last few bites. Now you can visually see those bites you would have taken not to be full, but rather because you felt obligated to clean your plate. Congratulations, you can actually measure your eating-smart achievement! Below are baby steps I took to achieve my goals.

## HOLLY'S HELPFUL HINTS TO CHANGE YOUR EATING

- Ended use of mayonnaise by moving to mustard, and then from mustard (which has salt) to fresh lemon or lime juice for flavor
- Eliminated prepared salad dressing by moving to watered-down, prepared dressing with vinegar, then to using vinegar sparingly, a squeeze of lemon, and a drizzle of olive oil
- Went from eating French bread carte blanche with oil, to only one piece of bread, to no bread at all, with the exception of a low-carb, low-sodium, multi-grain wrap
- Went from eating a cookie, to breaking the cookie in half and immediately throwing the other half in the trash, to not eating cookies and having an apple instead
- Went from eating packaged foods, to limiting packaged foods, to pre-cooking in bulk to mix and create healthy meals
- Went from leaving the house unprepared for potential hunger, resulting in eating out, to keeping a little lunchbox cooler in my car with healthy, fresh foods

- Eliminated using any spices containing sodium. There are lots of sodium-free spices available. Use fresh spices when possible
- Used a scale and a measuring cup to measure portion size until I got good at doing so visually
- Went from eating from any random plate at home to always eating from the same plate. This helps me to visually control my serving size
- Went from eating second servings to not going for seconds. I prepare my plate and put all the leftovers away immediately, before I eat, to avoid temptation for seconds
- Went from filling my plate with rice and potatoes, to filling plate with healthy, leafy greens
- Eliminated simple carbohydrates
- Went from leaving the house without water and getting dehydrated, to always leaving the house with a bottle of water and a piece of fruit just in case I got behind schedule

We all go off track. If you do, remember this: having one cookie doesn't mean you have to eat the entire jar.

Ground rules for success include not eating standing up at the kitchen counter. Eating standing up counts! Each time you go to put a handful of food in your mouth, grab a glass of water and drink. Keep a glass of water on the counter while you are making dinner. If you can't stomach plain water, try adding sliced cucumber, mint, or lemon or lime wedges. Sodium-free seltzer or green tea are other options.

Snacking while multi-tasking adds up to mindless overeating. Remind yourself to stay aware and avoid mindless snacking. All those little bites you take while preparing dinner easily add up to a meal. Naturally, you make yourself a plate and sit down to eat with the family. Think about what you have eaten during meal preparation. If you have been sampling while cooking, it is likely you're eating your meal before you actually sit down to eat your meal. Yes, that counts as eating twice. Overeating anything will make you pack on pounds. More calories in than calories out will equal weight gain.

Combating eating poorly during PMS is a challenge for every woman. As moms, it can really throw us off track due to raging hormones and resulting lack of patience for the kids. Mom is PMS-ing, and that blinking light in the kitchen is at red—DEFCON 5. Bloated, with aching boobs, and fighting cravings for salty and sugary foods, our temper is short. We feel extremely grouchy and sad, to the point where family members know our period is coming. The worst thing you can say to a mom who is PMS-ing is, "Mom is PMS-ing." Even though we are, that pisses us off even more. Everyone is supposed to pretend we are not moody and tip-toe lightly around us. Hardly! Premenstrual syndrome is a monthly headache for many of us. As we age, its symptoms often become even worse. Almost half of women experience moderate to severe PMS symptoms up to eleven days before their monthly period begins.

What you eat and drink can also have an effect on the severity of your symptoms. Studies indicate women with the highest intakes of calcium and vitamin D are less likely to develop PMS.[14] Calcium-rich foods on your eating plan include

[14] Cari Nierenberg, reviewed by Kathleen Zelman, "8 Diet Dos and Don'ts to Ease PMS," *WebMD*, n.d., http://www.webmd.com/women/pms/features/diet-and-pms?page=1

plain Greek yogurt, "no salt added" cottage cheese, and salmon. What about your cravings for chocolate and potato chips? PMS decreases the level of the feel-good chemical serotonin in the brain. These changes may affect a woman's mood. Chocolate makes you feel in love because it increases serotonin levels. Go for organic dark chocolate and limit your intake to one small piece. Take care of the craving before it gets out of control and you eat an entire box of chocolates.

Salt is another common craving resulting from serotonin reduction and seeking comfort in food. Salt is in almost everything already. Remember, approximately one teaspoon a day (1,200 milligrams) is all you are allowed. When you are already bloated from PMS, eliminate sodium from your eating, as it will only make your water retention worse. If you can't fight the salt craving, take a handful of pretzels and put the rest away. I also like to buy those little pre-measured snack bags to help me control my serving size. My secret for reducing bloating is to drink loads of water. You might wonder why I am telling you to drink more water when you are bloated. The extra water helps make the fluids in your blood less concentrated. This stimulates your body to release more water. I suggest water with sliced cucumber, lemon or lime wedges.

Cravings for salty and sweet foods while PMS-ing can easily add up to five hundred additional calories to your daily intake. Exercise is a great solution to PMS-ing. Working out helps reduce stress and increases those feel-good hormones in your brain. This result could help you control your cravings. Those extra calories you burn during exercise will keep your waistline in check. Being physically active not only keeps you lean and mean, it also reduces your symptoms of PMS. Tada!

# HOLLY'S LIST OF NATURAL, DIURETIC, LOW-CALORIE, LOW-SUGAR FOODS

- Unsweetened green tea
- Dandelion leaf
- Cucumber
- Asparagus
- Celery
- Garlic
- Horseradish
- Fresh kale leaf
- Musk melon
- Fresh ginger
- Blueberries
- Raw oats

Eating because of social pressure is another weight-loss hazard. Navigating the social parties and not overeating is a marathon in itself. Enter the dreaded holiday weight gain. How do you not indulge and manage to stay fit with all of those tempting buffets and passed hors d'oeuvres. We almost feel rude if we don't indulge. But choosing not to indulge is not rude, it is smart.

Prior to attending a social event where there will be food, avoid excess hunger. Do not let yourself become ravenously hungry by starving yourself for that special holiday event. Starving yourself causes your metabolism (caloric burn) to slow and results in overeating. Dress for success. Wear a form-fitting outfit that does not have any give. When you are full, your outfit will communicate the message to you because it will become tight feeling.

Beware of alcohol. Alcohol is nearly as calorically-dense as fat. Sip your cocktail slowly. Consider a glass of water between each cocktail. Drink lots of water. Flush out your system, feel full, and keep your skin clear. Hunger can often be mistaken for thirst. Drink a glass of water prior to eating.

At the event, choose foods that represent how you want your body to look. Do you want to look like a celery stick or a scallop wrapped in bacon? Think sexy as you choose your foods. They should reflect your ultimate body image. When selecting a dessert, immediately half the portion size. If you take one slice of cake, cut it in two and take half. Throw away the other half before you are tempted to eat it.

Finally, be sure to mingle among the guests. The more you are mingling and chatting, the less time you will have to put food in your mouth. Avoid being trapped in a corner with your best friend, scarfing down your favorite holiday foods. Meet some new people. After all, you are attending the event to socialize, not to eat.

# 15

# Savvy Chef

*Hollyism: "Preparedness is key to success."*

Why is it that no matter how many times we perform this morning routine, it is still like a dress rehearsal? My two sons are seated at the breakfast table, I whip open the cereal cabinet, and rush past the fridge, grabbing the milk and orange juice. I set the milk down on the table and pour the orange juice into their cups, only to head back and yell at my daughter to get out of bed before she makes everyone late. In a craze, I run back into the kitchen and around the corner to slam, head first, into the kitchen cereal cabinet I had left wide open. I literally fall to the floor with an egg swelling on my temple. While I lie there, trying to regain consciousness, I hear my son's voice calling from the kitchen table, "Mom, where is my cereal?"

Kids finally out the door, I realize how hungry I am; in the morning chaos, I have had no time to eat. Glancing at the leftovers on the kitchen table, I experience a moment of indecision: do I eat the half-eaten bowl of Captain Crunch, or the quarter piece of strawberry Pop Tart? The uneaten crust of the French toast with butter, or the fragment of pancake drenched in syrup? It is time to clean out the kitchen cabinets and remove temptation for an unhealthy, quick-fix breakfast. Our children have incredible metabolisms, and in the challenge to get them to eat breakfast, we resort to accommodating their palate. As Mom, in order to be healthy, we have to think healthy for our family.

Plan ahead nutritionally by asking yourself, "Is this food a good choice for me?" If the answer is no, why would you feed it to your children? Children need to be exposed to a new food over a two-week period—sometimes up to eleven or more times—in order for them to acclimate to taste and texture. Put healthy foods in front of them time and time again. When tasting a new food, my daughter says, "Mom, my taste buds aren't that open." To open your children's taste buds to a new food, pair it with a familiar food for a friendly introduction. Most critically, your children should see you eating the food you are requesting they eat. As a result, when you are grazing on leftover breakfast, it will be abundant with healthy options. Munching on high-fat breakfast options like sausage, bacon, and cheese will run you the risk of craving even more junk food during the day. Processed foods don't do a good job of keeping your body fueled and always leave you wanting more. Think of it as your beautiful, natural body not recognizing a foreign substance. It is extremely important to eat breakfast for weight loss and maintenance. Make sure you pay attention to the content and quality of what you eat.

Include protein in your breakfast. The longest period of muscle breakdown is while you sleep. Protein fuels muscle, which is critical to good health. You don't have to categorize foods between breakfast and other meals. Breakfast or mid-day snack foods are important staples to have on hand at any time of day. I have eaten leftover fish or chicken as part of my breakfast. Don't be afraid to eat what you crave. If the clock tells you it is time for eggs or oatmeal, but your tummy tells you it wants the leftover chicken breast, abide by your tummy.

I find that during the day, most people are able to show discipline in the foods they consume. Evening is the time where most go way off their eating plan. Family multitasking and stress can take a mom away from eating awareness. What mom hasn't reached to text another in desperation at the dinner witching hour, only to get the reply, "Going nuts here too. Someone save us!" It is that early evening dinnertime hour when the kids and mom are equally exhausted. Ask yourself if you will you even taste those cookies, given how fast you are going to shove them down your throat. The faster you eat them, the less it counts, right? If nobody sees you, no calories in! Nothing worthwhile is easy, and you and your hot body are worth your very best effort. Here is the hot mommy plan of attack.

"What's for dinner, Mom?" The most-asked question, second only to, "Are we there yet?" The "as long as my children are happy" mentality no longer applies at dinnertime. Is your kitchen in a restaurant or your home? You are certainly not the house wait staff! Limit choices for your family and your sanity. Prepare the basics so you can create multiple meals from various ingredients. I am not telling you your kids should not eat healthy. But are they going to eat the huge salad you are? Hell, no! This is actually one area where it is easy to keep everyone happy.

Pre-prepare yourself for ease and flexibility at dinnertime. Eating healthy requires preparedness. You wouldn't start your day not knowing your schedule, would you? Why allow your eating to be random? I have a cooking day twice per week. On that day, I cook huge family servings of chicken breasts, lean pork tenderloin, fresh turkey breast, salmon, and lightly-steamed veggies. I literally do not cook again for at least three days. Not cooking every day will save you from snacking, as you taste your dishes while preparing. It will also make your life much more efficient to cook in bulk by simply throwing together dishes from prepared foods. Having pre-pared food on hand will prevent you from that last minute decision to order take-out food. Use your pre-prepared ingredients to create a variety of delectable dishes.

Will there be nights where you allow your children grilled cheese, chicken fingers, or macaroni and cheese? Of course. That doesn't make you a bad nutritional mom, it just makes you normal. If you can't deal with making the kids' plates without eating the crust you cut off the grilled cheese, please try and eat your dinner first. Make yourself a plate, grab a big glass of water, and EAT. This strategy will curb your appetite. Your hands will not be shaking with desire as you load their plates with gooey macaroni and cheese. Mommy torture! Just picture that macaroni and cheese on your thighs and you will stop your fork before it reaches your mouth. The likelihood of your children starving because you took fifteen minutes to eat your dinner first is highly unlikely. They will survive. So eat before you overeat!

You survived dinnertime and are now clearing the dishes. If your children are old enough, teach them to clear their own plates. Food in the trash and dishes in the sink or on the counter, whichever they can reach. I know it is more time-efficient for you to clear them, but not waist-wise. Your children will learn responsibility early, and you will not be tempted to clean their plates by snacking on their leftovers. Ask yourself, as you are eating the bites of leftover chicken nuggets, "Am I the mom or the family pet?" We are all wired to clean our plates and the plates of our offspring. If you have ever had a dog, it's an easy equation. Dogs eat scraps. Picture your face in a dog bowl chomping down those scraps. A cute collar studded with crystals around your neck with a dog tag hanging that says, "Mom." It's not pretty, but your body will be if you avoid scrap eating. That's worth the mental image!

To create an efficient eating strategy for you and your family, choose a main ingredient that you have cooked in bulk, like meat, fish, poultry, or a vegetarian staple. From that ingredient, create your Hot Mommy's Dinner Menu. Mix and match base ingredients to create dinner for you, kids, and hubby to make everyone fun, happy meals.

Before going shopping, make a list for the grocery store so you are not tempted to buy more than you need. Take home good food by shopping fresh. Fresh items are typically found on the outside aisles of the grocery store. Those are the aisles that require refrigeration. The inside aisles are primarily packed with processed food that has preservatives. Shopping the outside aisles will bring amazing results. The grocery store is a major excursion when you bring baby along and can be a stressful errand. Aisle upon aisle, your child keeps grabbing random items off the shelves while you keep putting them back. I am a big fan of the people who actually push the cute cart that looks like a carnival ride.

Before you grab a bag of potato chips and start shoving them in your mouth due to stress, take a deep breath. We have all been there as moms; you are not alone. Remember that as you pass the woman in the aisle that gives you the understanding "I have been there" look, smile as your child is having a baby breakdown.

## WHAT'S ON HOLLY'S SHOPPING LIST?

- Unsweetened green tea (iced or hot)
- Plain, non-fat Greek yogurt
- Fruit: berries, bananas, apples
- Lemons and limes (for cooking)
- Flaxseed
- Chia seed
- Plain oatmeal
- Liquid egg whites
- Eggs
- Chicken breasts
- Turkey breasts (whole)
- Salmon
- Spinach
- Low-fat feta or 2 percent shredded cheddar cheese
- Skim milk or skim almond milk
- Cinnamon (hot spices increase metabolism)

**Note:** Unsweetened green tea is an appetite suppressant and increases metabolism, which is the rate at which you burn calories.

# 16

# Happy Mommy, Happy Home

*Hollyism: "Being a mom makes you more important—not less—so prioritize you're well-being."*

Being a mom is a lifetime journey. Time will fly, and suddenly, your newborn baby will be in fourth grade and you will barely be able to figure out their homework. They won't hesitate to let you know that you are a complete artifact because they don't do math like math was done when you were a kid. Forget about the guilt for missing the school morning reading event your child would have participated in for five minutes, yet would have caused you to miss three hours of other obligations. Trust me, you weren't the only mom who wasn't present. At home or outside the home, *every mom is a working mom.*

Dreaded middle school drama enters far too early. In this generation, due to our food chain, early puberty is rampant. My nine-year-old daughter is sprouting breasts and acting like she is sixteen. Experts say that on average, puberty is starting earlier in the United States than it has in the past—sometimes as early as age nine. Not more than one girl with PMS allowed in the household at a time.

Next is high school where your children know everything about everything. You know nothing and owe them an explanation for everything you know that they haven't yet learned. Your daughter pilfers your makeup, clothes, and handbags, and your teenage son needs to take extremely long showers.

Driver's license terror leads to late nights again. No sleep, but not from waking for nighttime feeding, but because your darling is out late and driving. Anxiously, you wait up to hear the house door open and feel relief that they are home safe. Or you hear the cell phone ring, which means they are deviously avoiding curfew and parental confrontation. Oh, the frustration.

When the kids go to college or move away from home, separation anxiety and empty nest syndrome ultimately descend. I suggest you turn your nest into an erotic sex chamber, complete with a pole for dancing to literally create a virtual strip-away stress sanctuary. Bondage, toys, mirrors—whatever makes you happy. Recreate you!

By reading this book, I hope you feel empowered at whatever stage of fitness you are at today to progress to your personal goal. Permission is granted to gracefully decline to partake in the mom-petition. Motherhood is about you—physically, mentally, and emotionally. Only you are capable of knowing what form of health and fitness suits your lifestyle.

You are armed with all the secret weapons that you need to drop those extra mommy pounds. Even if you haven't started to make one change in your eating or exercise, please congratulate yourself on reading this book and being aware that you want to make a change. Exhale with the knowledge that you are not alone in mommy-hood. Embrace your support village and your diligent effort to lose weight and get fit. The keys are now yours; use them to unlock your potential.

Approach each day with an open mind and a sense of humor. Laughing at ourselves releases stress and is great for strengthening our abs. Fitness and eating smart are not complicated. You must have the sheer tenacity to stick with it. Failure is the instrument of success. You will have bad days and good days. You will lose five pounds and gain back three. Learn from mistakes and look forward, using them to strategize the next day. Use your journal to document and review your good days and your bad. You are a mom, but you are still a human. Think of yourself with the same love and patience that you do your children.

## AN ANECDOTAL DAY IN THE LIFE OF HOT MOMMY

Another hectic day fitting in exercise, eating smart, and a million other things mere mortals can't fathom, but moms manage to accomplish. Your husband/partner keeps texting you to meet for hot sex during lunch hour. Decisions, decisions. You grab a quick shower and slide on your jeans that fit just right.

On the way out the door, you notice ten things you didn't get done today and get side tracked. You are late to pick up your kids at school *again*. It is raining, and in your hectic rush out the door you forgot to grab an umbrella. As you arrive at school a sense of calmness descends and the sidewalk rises to meet you.

The squeaking of your soaking wet shoes syncs to the beat of your favorite song. Happily you gather your children smiling to yourself, unbothered by the rain. Your hair and clothes are drenched, reflecting a radiant fashion statement of strength.

Other moms think you surely forgot your umbrella on purpose because, well, you are that "Hot Mom" and you are comfortable with yourself. The mommy who once made you feel insecure is no longer significant. Now sitting in your car, windshield wipers in the same torrential downpour as when our book began...now the same wipers peacefully sweep back and forth. You glance in the rearview mirror at your beautiful children and smile. It hasn't been an easy journey, but they are worth it and so are you.

*You are at your personal best!*
*Congratulations!*